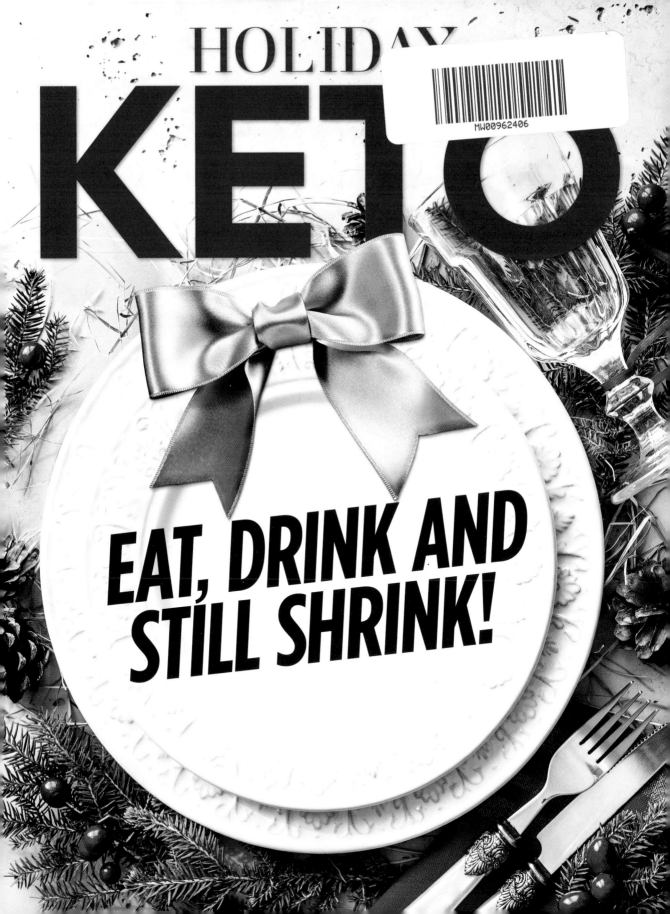

HOLIDAY KETO

EAT, DRINK AND STILL SHRINK!

HOLIDAY KETO

EAT, DRINK AND STILL SHRINK!

BY MICHELLE STACEY

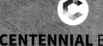

CENTENNIAL BOOKS

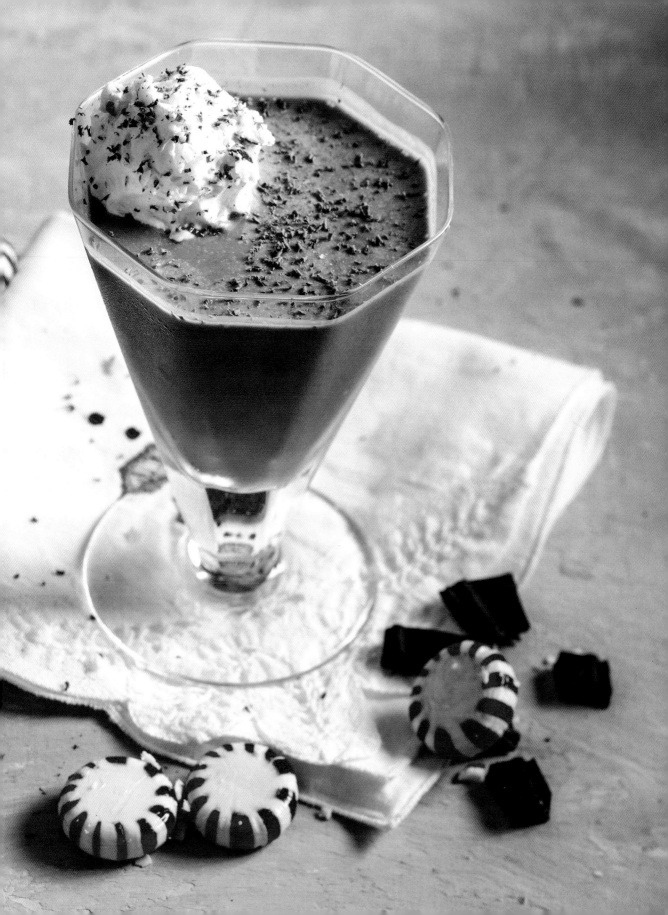

Contents

156

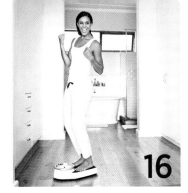
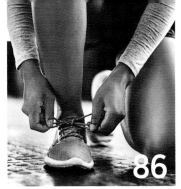
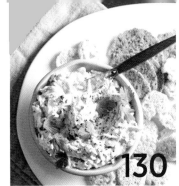

CHAPTER 1

THE BASICS

08 Why Keto?
The reasons it has become a way of life for many.

16 The Science Behind the Diet
How keto changes you.

20 Keto's Hidden Benefits
The plan's potential health boosts are far reaching.

28 Fats vs. Carbs
Why you should favor one over the other.

36 Best Oils
Savory staples for better health—and flavor.

38 Keto in Terms of Food
You may be surprised at what you *can* eat.

44 Coping With the Side Effects
How to deal with the diet's early-stage downsides.

50 Glossary: Keto Lingo
The vocab you need to follow the plan.

54 Get Organized
Restock your pantry and reframe your mind.

CHAPTER 2

SEASONAL STRATEGIES

62 Survive the Season
Stay strong amid the many holiday temptations.

68 Table for One
How to stick to your plan when it's time to party.

72 Eating Out? No Problem
Easy ways to stay on your diet when away from home.

78 The Cycle Plan
This way of eating makes it easy to outlast the season.

82 "Oops, I Ate It!"
Bounce back when you've broken your own rules.

86 The Stay-Fit Holiday Plan
Give yourself the gift of fitness when things get nuts.

92 Ready, Set, Goals!
Discover the tools to make your plan a success.

98 What's Sleep Got to Do With It?
There's more to shut-eye than feeling refreshed.

102 Drink Up!
Water is a key part of transitioning to keto.

106 Easy Entertaining
Take the stress out of holiday hosting with simple tips.

116 How Much to Make?
Guidelines to make sure everyone feels satisfied.

CHAPTER 3

RECIPES

120 Beverages
Raise a glass with these keto-friendly cocktails that will be the hit of your holiday party.

130 Appetizers
Kick off the festivities with keto-approved finger foods that look fancy but are a cinch to make.

140 Salads
These starters are filled with flavor and are always dressed to impress.

148 Soups
Hearty bowls like these are the perfect way to warm up on a cool day.

156 Entrées
Elegant but easy main courses that are certain to draw rave reviews whenever they are served.

166 Sides
An array of crowd-pleasing dishes that are surprisingly low in carbohydrates.

176 Desserts
End things on a sweet note with low-sugar recipes that taste indulgent but totally fit your keto lifestyle.

186 Index

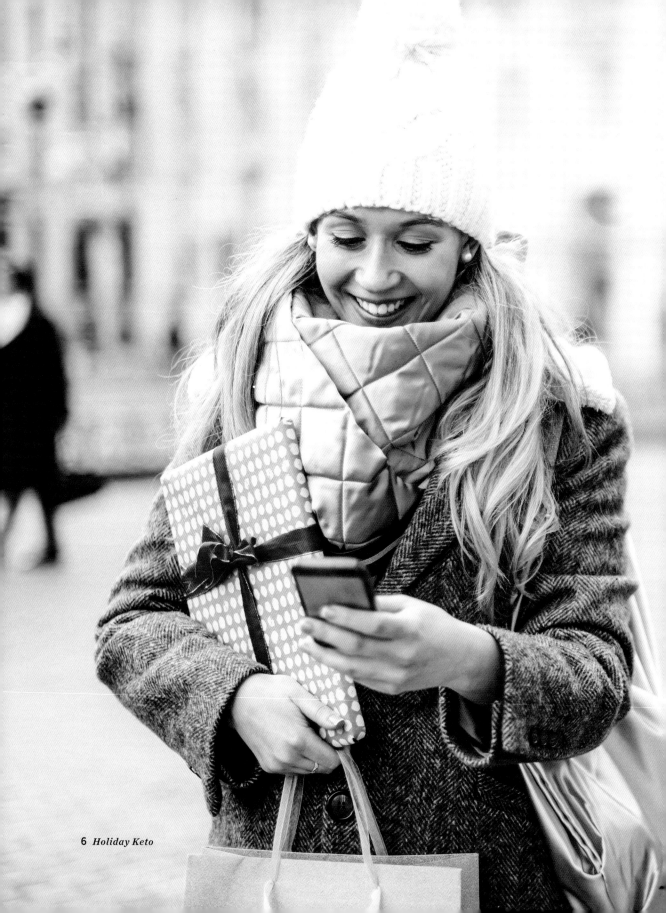

Chapter 1

The Basics

LEARN THE FUNDAMENTALS OF AMERICA'S FAVORITE DIET.

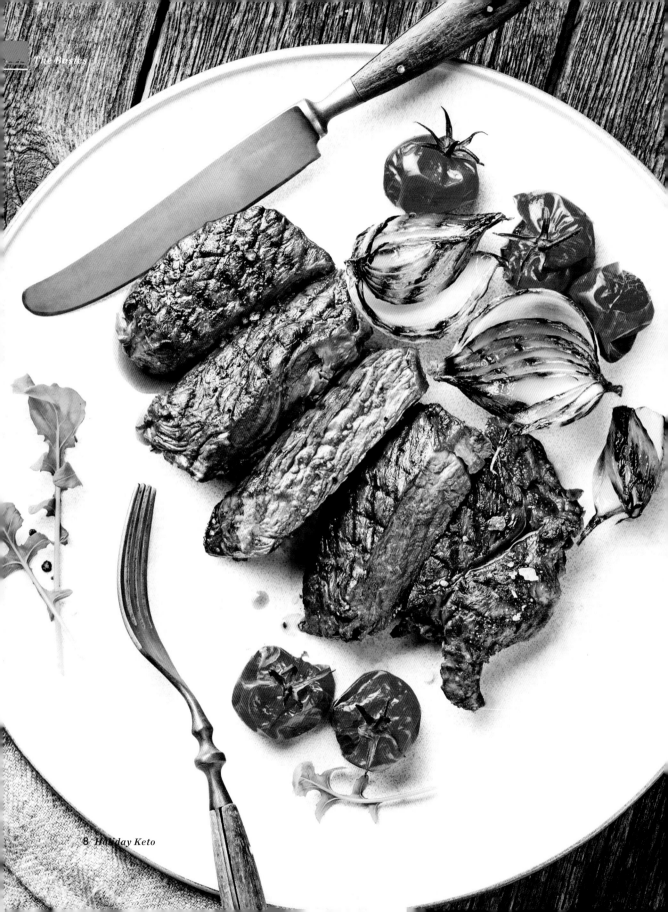

Why Keto?

The ketogenic lifestyle is the fastest-growing diet on the planet. **Here's how it works—and what lies behind its success.**

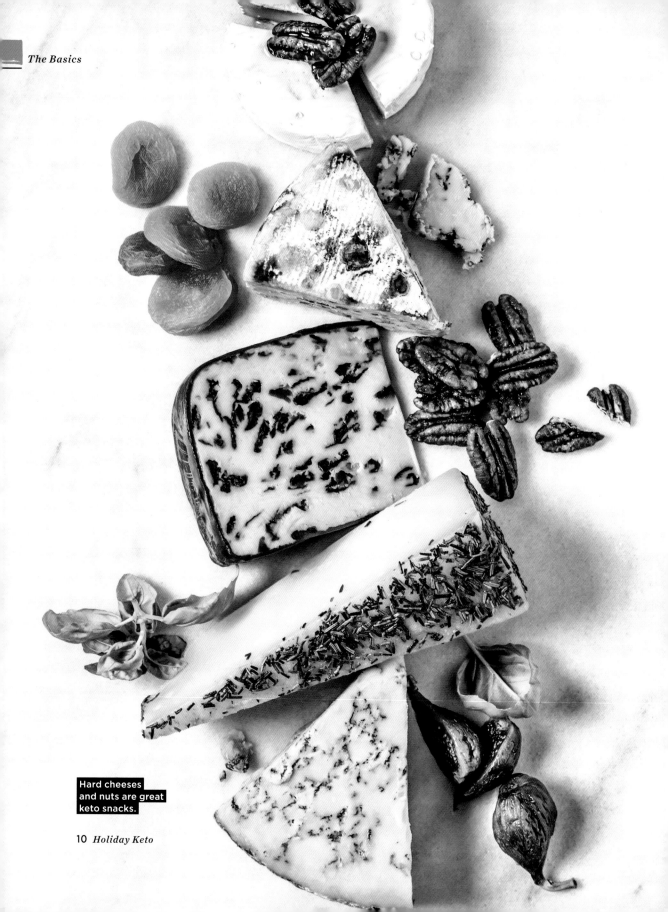

Hard cheeses and nuts are great keto snacks.

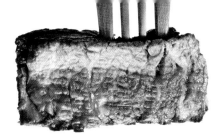

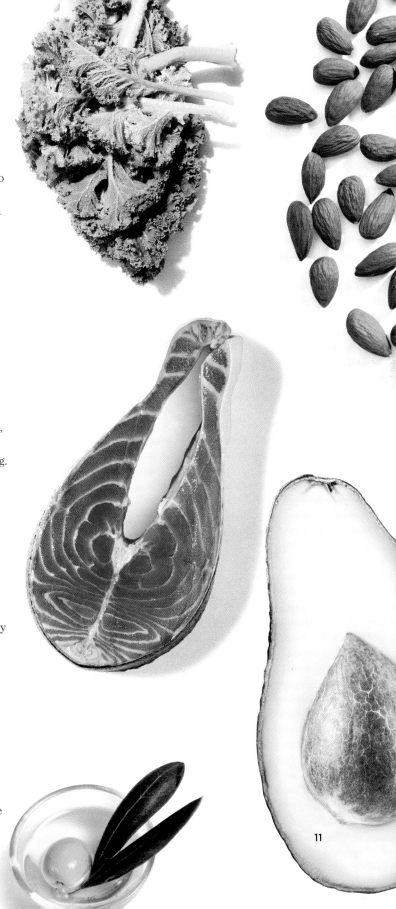

I f you don't know at least one person who is "doing keto"—a friend, a sister, an uncle, a Facebook friend from your high school class—you may be in a minority these days. Fad diets have been with us for more than a century, but few, if any, have had as meteoric a rise as the ketogenic diet, popularly known as keto. In January 2016, Google searches for "keto" were barely a blip on the analytics radar; by the end of 2018, keto had far outstripped the competition (including the popular paleo, Whole30 and intermittent-fasting plans) to become the most searched-for diet of that year—by a mile. In 2018, five of the top 10 Google diet searches were for keto foods, including keto pancakes, keto cheesecake and keto cookies. And the trend keeps going.

So of course, those of us who haven't yet tried it are wondering: *Should I have what they're having?*

Along with: *What's the allure of this diet, anyway?* First off, keto is a hugely Instagram-friendly diet, with #keto boasting more than 17 million posts. The success stories are everywhere, including celebrities Khloé Kardashian, Tim Tebow and Halle Berry. Another draw is that many people report feeling less hunger on keto, even while they're losing weight.

Meanwhile, a steady flow of studies has turned up increasingly solid findings for keto. A 2019 report from the National Institutes of Health (NIH) concluded that "a very-low-carbohydrate and high-fat ketogenic diet" has been "proven to be very effective for rapid weight loss." Other research, in both humans and lab animals, has shown that keto may help many people manage blood sugar levels, prevent or treat metabolic syndrome (a precursor to type 2 diabetes), reduce cardiovascular risk factors, reduce inflammation in the body (a major cause of disease), and even promote energy and mental clarity. That evidence has helped push keto further into the mainstream, and in the summer of 2018 a group of 10 physicians went to Washington, D.C., to extol low-carb diets to the Dietary Guidelines for Americans advisory committee, urging members to include them in the 2020 protocols.

How Keto Works

The key to keto is that it induces your body to switch its fuel source, explains Josh Axe, D.N.M., the founder of *draxe.com* and the author of *Keto Diet*. "Rather than relying on counting calories, limiting portion sizes or requiring lots of willpower, keto works by burning fat for energy instead of burning glucose." When you switch from eating a standard American diet—which the NIH estimates gets 55 percent of its calories from carbs—to a keto plan of at most 5 to 10 percent from carbs, that changes how your whole system operates.

Carbs are quickly broken down into sugar, or glucose, once you eat them. They are your body's favorite fuel, because they turn so easily into energy. But that also means that whatever energy you don't need right then is just as easily moved into storage, in the form of fat cells. The body's alternative fuel source is fats, but they're harder to break down, so they're used only when you run out of glucose. By reducing your carb intake to near-zero on keto, you force your body to run on fat instead. It does that both by using fat to fuel your muscles, and by sending dietary fats to your liver to be turned into chemicals called ketones (hence the name of the diet),

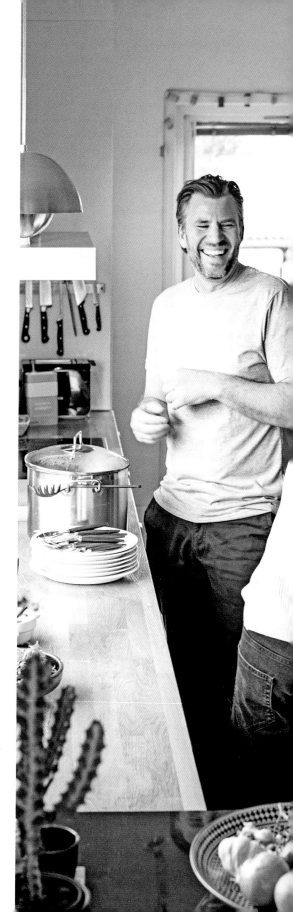

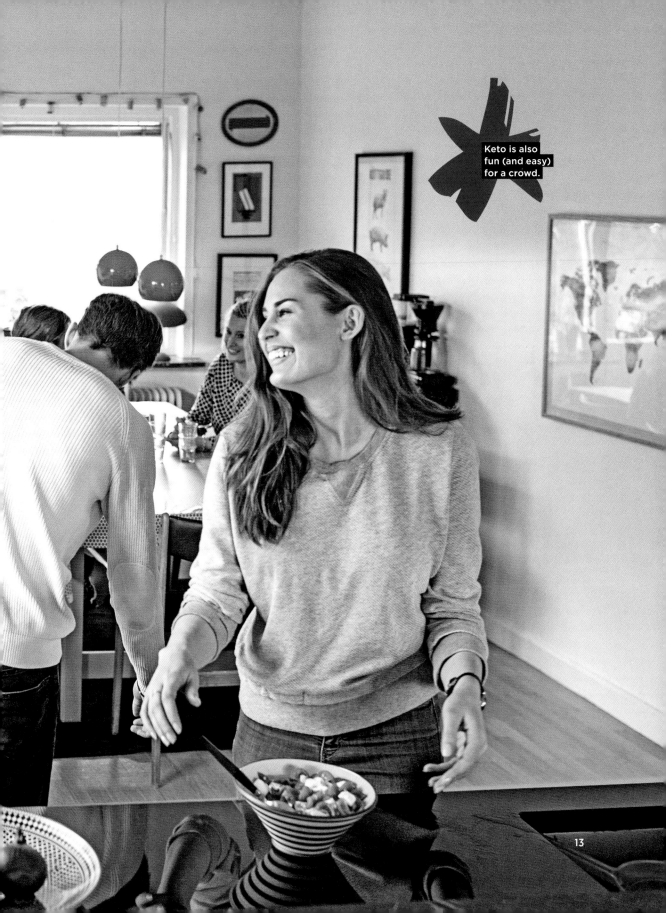

Keto is also fun (and easy) for a crowd.

13

a third source of fuel for your cells. Ketones are important, says Andreas Eenfeldt, M.D., founder of the online Diet Doctor program, because "the brain consumes lots of energy every day, but unlike the muscles it can't run on fat directly. It can only run on either glucose or ketones."

If you restrict your carb intake for long enough—from a few days to a few weeks—you enter ketosis, in which your body is burning mostly fat. And that's not just the fats you are eating, but also stored body fat, when needed. So rather than storing more energy in fat cells, as you would on a carb-based diet, you'll be taking fat out of storage and burning it off. The result: weight loss, along with other benefits that may result from avoiding carbs, including lowering inflammation and steadying your blood sugar levels.

Getting to Ketosis

Prompting your body into ketosis involves a fairly simple equation with three variables: the macronutrients fats, protein and carbs. "A rough guideline is about 5 to 10 percent of energy from carbohydrates—the fewer carbs, the more effective—15 to 20 percent from protein, and around 75 percent from fat," says Eenfeldt. It's not complicated, he adds; it boils down to avoiding too many carbs. An easy way to do that is to think of carbohydrate intake in terms of grams, staying under 50 grams per day, and ideally below 20 grams. As an example, a bagel has 48 grams of carbs, putting it off-limits for someone on keto.

Two tablespoons of cream cheese on that bagel, in contrast, have only 1.2 grams of carbs. That helps explain the basic approach to keto: You don't have to worry about the numbers as much as the types of food you're eating, and the ones you're not. On keto, you eat lots of high-fat foods—meats, fatty fish, olive oil, butter, avocados—and avoid high-carb foods like breads, sweets and starchy vegetables (see "Key Keto Food Facts," at right).

But Is It Safe?

It's not surprising that after decades of government advice promoting a low-fat diet, some people have this question. So far, the vast majority of studies show an array of benefits and few risks, although scientists point out we do not yet have very long-term studies to confirm that. "I wouldn't say there are no risks, but the risks are relatively low," says Elizabeth Parks, Ph.D., a professor of nutrition and exercise physiology at the University of Missouri School of Medicine. "If you are relatively healthy, it is not a dangerous diet to try, and many people find it sustainable. If you're diabetic, however, you should check with your doctor before you start, because some diabetes medicines do not work well on keto." Indeed, anyone embarking on keto should check with their doctor, just in case.

The healthfulness of keto also depends on how you carry it out. A high-fat diet could be full of foods like bacon, sausage, pork rinds and fast food, none of which are very healthy. Some people do take that approach, known as "dirty keto," but it's not ideal and won't convey the same benefits as "clean keto." "Processed foods can cause inflammation, poor gut health, allergies, fluid retention and hormonal issues," says Axe. "Those all can make weight loss more difficult." One more thing, says Parks: Take a multivitamin to cover your bases.

Says one keto dieter who lost 100 pounds: "I feel so great now, I'll never go back."

Meet Meats! They may become your favorite foods on keto.

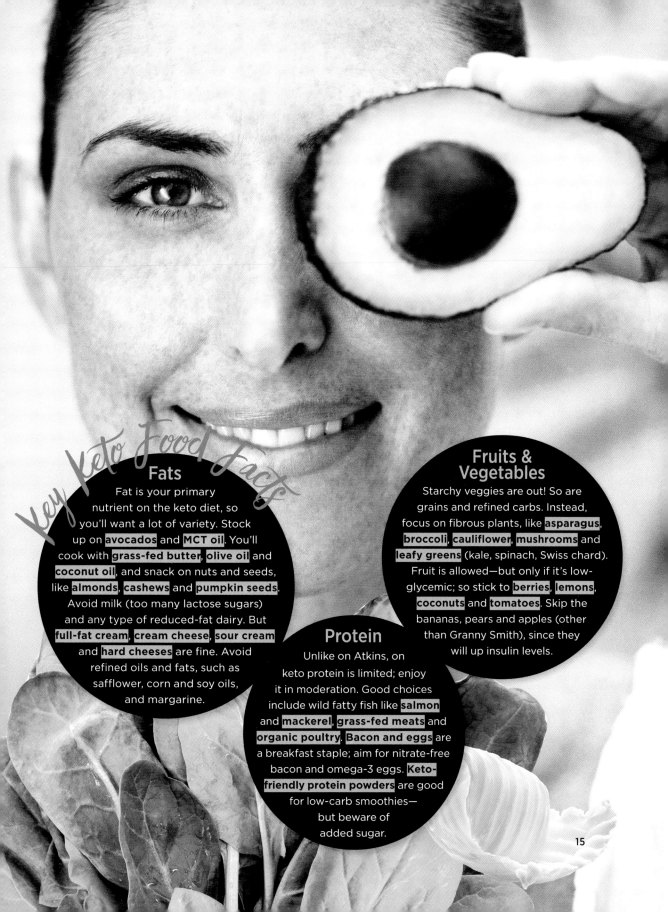

Key Keto Food Facts

Fats

Fat is your primary nutrient on the keto diet, so you'll want a lot of variety. Stock up on **avocados** and **MCT oil**. You'll cook with **grass-fed butter**, **olive oil** and **coconut oil**, and snack on nuts and seeds, like **almonds**, **cashews** and **pumpkin seeds**. Avoid milk (too many lactose sugars) and any type of reduced-fat dairy. But **full-fat cream**, **cream cheese**, **sour cream** and **hard cheeses** are fine. Avoid refined oils and fats, such as safflower, corn and soy oils, and margarine.

Fruits & Vegetables

Starchy veggies are out! So are grains and refined carbs. Instead, focus on fibrous plants, like **asparagus**, **broccoli**, **cauliflower**, **mushrooms** and **leafy greens** (kale, spinach, Swiss chard). Fruit is allowed—but only if it's low-glycemic; so stick to **berries**, **lemons**, **coconuts** and **tomatoes**. Skip the bananas, pears and apples (other than Granny Smith), since they will up insulin levels.

Protein

Unlike on Atkins, on keto protein is limited; enjoy it in moderation. Good choices include wild fatty fish like **salmon** and **mackerel**, **grass-fed meats** and **organic poultry**. **Bacon and eggs** are a breakfast staple; aim for nitrate-free bacon and omega-3 eggs. **Keto-friendly protein powders** are good for low-carb smoothies— but beware of added sugar.

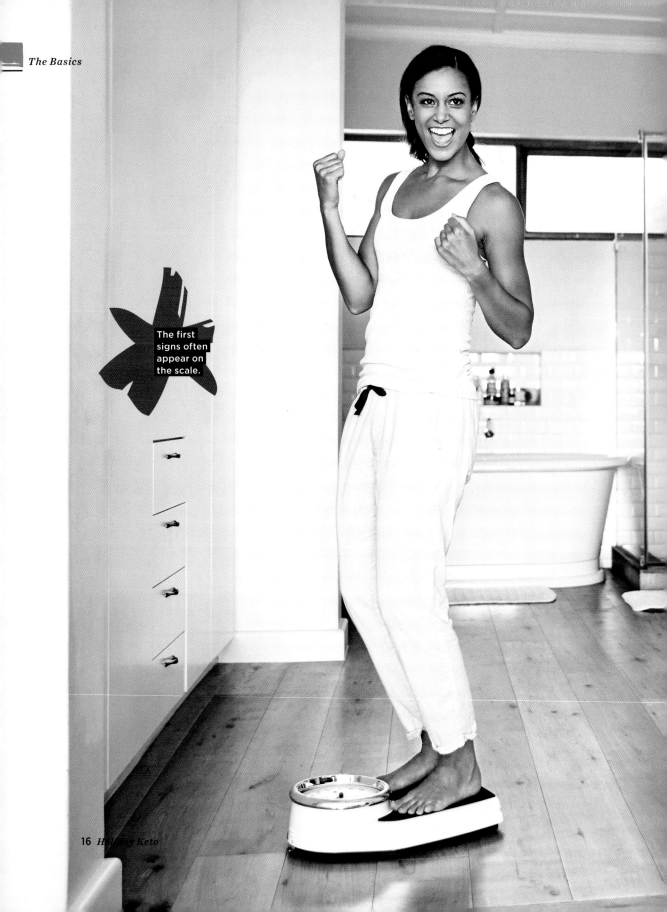

The first signs often appear on the scale.

THE Science BEHIND THE DIET

Learn the inside story of **how keto changes your body's habits**—for the better.

The first and most obvious effect of keto is weight loss. But the mechanisms that contribute to that outcome are at work far beneath what you see in the mirror, down at the cellular level. And at the heart of it all are the complicated actions of carbohydrates. They are nature's easy food, quickly transformed into energy. But the nature of our "food universe" has shifted so much since the caveman days that carbs have become a nemesis. Here's how keto changes that.

Carbs, Meet Insulin

The hormone insulin, manufactured by the pancreas, is a powerhouse. It is also carbs' enabler. When you eat carbs, the natural sugars they contain crowd into your blood, but they can't get directly into your cells, raising blood sugar levels. Insulin, released by the pancreas, acts as the "key" to shunt sugar (glucose) into cells, bringing blood sugar back down to normal while giving you an energy boost. If there's more sugar than your cells need, insulin stores the leftovers in fat cells.

It's a neat little system—unless you eat too many carbs, especially highly processed sugary foods and refined grains that quickly break down. These cause a spike in blood sugar, in turn prompting a high rush of insulin. "Too much insulin forces our fat cells into calorie-storage overdrive," says David Ludwig, M.D., professor of nutrition at Harvard's T.H. Chan School of Public Health. "These rapidly growing fat cells then hoard too many calories, leaving too few for the rest of the body, so we get hungry again." Then we eat again, and store even more calories. In the past few decades, as experts pushed low-fat diets, consumption of simple carbs skyrocketed, along with obesity rates.

Enter Fats

When you replace carbs with fats and some protein, that scenario changes drastically. Your body can use fats directly, so there's no need for insulin to open your cells. The fats in a keto diet function as a "clean fuel," burning steadily without sugar highs and lows, so you don't have the hunger spikes. And because insulin locks carbs into storage, when their intake drops, those "storage areas" open up. "When insulin levels go very low, fat-burning increases," explains Andreas Eenfeldt, M.D., founder of Diet Doctor. "You can access and burn your fat stores."

The ketones are the other "secret sauce" of keto. After you cut carbs, some of the fat

Waist Loss
Keto targets abdominal fat—the most deadly kind..

you eat goes to the liver to be turned into ketones, alternative-fuel molecules for your body. Fat is a good fuel, but ketones are especially efficient and easily accessed. And your brain uses only two fuels—glucose and ketones.

Why the Weight Loss?

Dropping pounds is only one of the benefits of keto, but for many people it is the impetus to start the diet. The mechanisms of weight loss appear to be multipronged, according to Harvard's School of Public Health. First, fat is more satiating than carbs, because it leaves the stomach more slowly and doesn't cause the highs and lows that prompt hunger. Studies also show keto may tamp down the release of the "hunger hormone," ghrelin. People who lost weight on keto had lower levels of ghrelin in their blood, even though most dieters tend to have *more* of the hormone (a possible reason for yo-yo weight regain).

An increase in metabolism—the rate at which your body burns calories—may also aid keto weight loss. A recent clinical study by Ludwig, among the largest, most rigorous "feeding trials" ever conducted, found that overweight adults who cut carbs and replaced them with fat burned 250 calories more per day than people who ate a high-carb, low-fat diet; some burned as many as 400 calories more. This helps explain why most people who lose weight on a low-fat diet gain it back; it has been shown that dieting lowers metabolism. Keto seems to do the opposite, helping you burn more fat while still feeling satiated. Has science finally found the perfect diet?

The Macronutrient Ratios of Keto

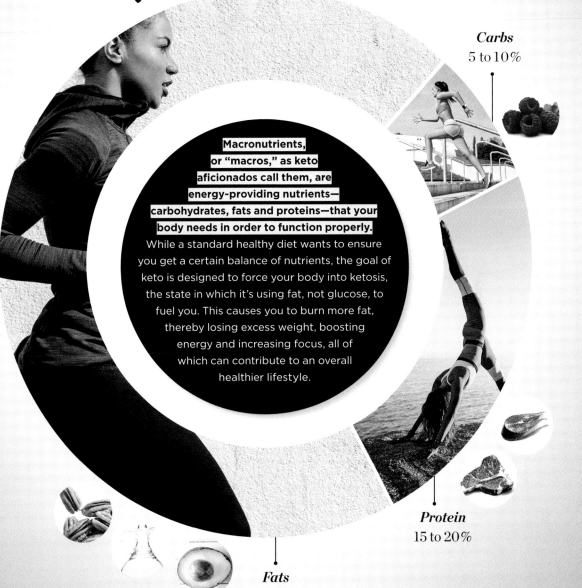

Macronutrients, or "macros," as keto aficionados call them, are energy-providing nutrients—carbohydrates, fats and proteins—that your body needs in order to function properly. While a standard healthy diet wants to ensure you get a certain balance of nutrients, the goal of keto is designed to force your body into ketosis, the state in which it's using fat, not glucose, to fuel you. This causes you to burn more fat, thereby losing excess weight, boosting energy and increasing focus, all of which can contribute to an overall healthier lifestyle.

Carbs
5 to 10%

Protein
15 to 20%

Fats
75%

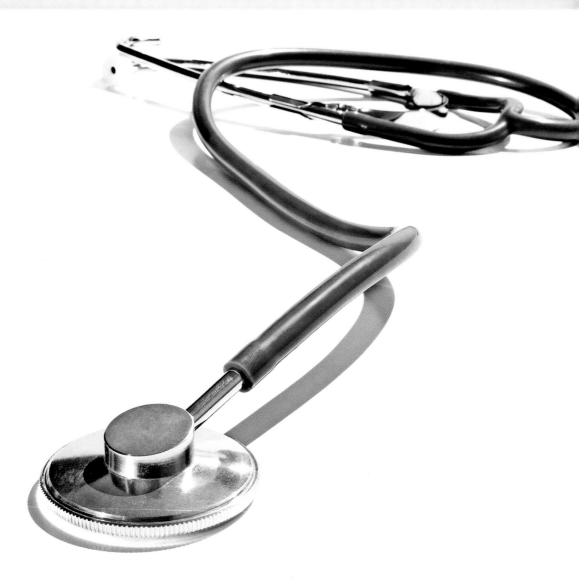

KETO'S
Hidden
Benefits

The diet's quick weight loss is what drives the Instagram clicks, **but the potential health boosts are more than skin deep.**

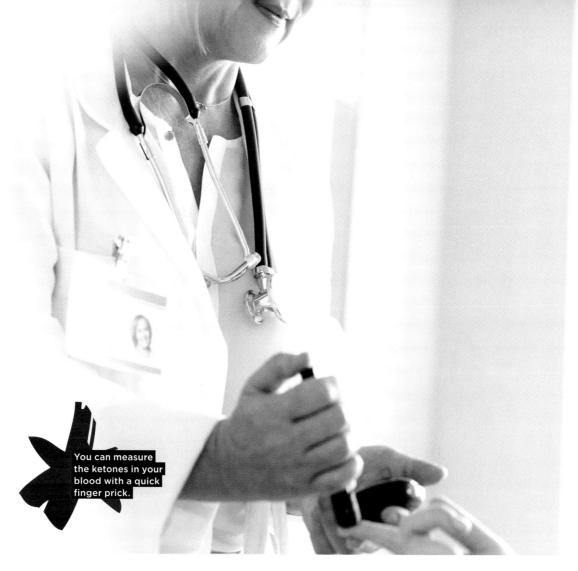

You can measure the ketones in your blood with a quick finger prick.

The promise of dropping pounds while not feeling hungry is what entices many dieters to try keto for the first time. Once they start, though, they find other health incentives to stick to it—often to their surprise. Those with insulin resistance or type 2 diabetes may see their blood sugar levels start to stabilize; people who are worried about heart disease can see cardiovascular-risk markers, like triglycerides and high blood pressure, improve.

Mounting evidence is showing possible benefits throughout the body, and even a usually conservative government source like the National Institutes of Health (NIH) is now acknowledging "promising results" in studies of keto's effect on neurological problems and metabolic disorders. Here, a head-to-toe breakdown of the good keto can do in your body.

Brain

The connection between brain function and keto goes back nearly a century, when neurologists treating epilepsy patients who didn't respond to medication found that if they fasted for two or three days

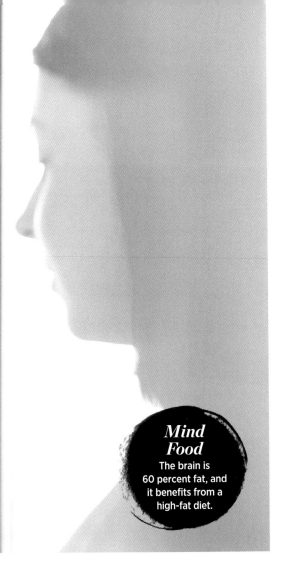

Mind Food

The brain is 60 percent fat, and it benefits from a high-fat diet.

some people are reporting this as a side benefit," says Weiss. He adds that he has been on the keto diet for a year and feels "terrific"—including having a new kind of mental energy.

What causes the connection? One theory is that by reducing sugar intake to almost nil, the keto diet reduces inflammation throughout the body (sugar has been shown to be inflammatory). Many neurological conditions, including Alzheimer's, have been linked to inflammation, so calming it down in the brain could have far-reaching effects. Another possibility is that ketones may be a superior fuel for the brain, which can utilize only glucose or ketones (not fat directly) for energy. A study in the journal *Transactions of the American Clinical and Climatological Association* found that the principal ketone produced by the liver, D-beta-hydroxybutyrate, is "not just a fuel but a 'superfuel'—more efficiently producing ATP [the body's primary energy carrier] than either glucose or fatty acid." Scientists working with neuron (brain) cells in the laboratory have found that this ketone protected the cells against exposure to toxins associated with Alzheimer's or Parkinson's, both neurodegenerative diseases. This may be why some studies have shown that ketosis enhances memory in people with mild cognitive impairment.

Heart

Although there has not been a long-term, clinical study of heart-health outcomes while following the keto diet, there is abundant evidence that keto helps many people improve their "markers" for heart disease. These include risk factors like high blood pressure, high triglycerides, low HDL cholesterol (the "good" kind), and high

(which makes the liver produce ketones), their seizures went away. Before long, doctors realized that producing ketones by withdrawing almost all carbohydrates from the diet had the same effect—and was easier to accomplish, especially in children. These days, many keto dieters talk about feeling a mental clarity once they're in ketosis, notes Ethan Weiss, M.D., an associate professor at the Cardiovascular Research Institute at the University of California, San Francisco. "While I haven't seen any rigorous trials measuring 'clarity,' and I'm not suggesting people go on the diet simply for that reason, blood glucose levels. Studies suggest that many of the heart-health benefits may be driven, first and foremost, by the weight loss, which is beneficial to your arteries and also helps reduce inflammation (which can drive heart disease). "From my perspective as a cardiologist, if my patients lose a bunch of weight and are feeling better, and their metabolism, glucose levels and insulin sensitivity all get better, at least we can say we're not increasing their chance of having a heart attack," says Weiss. "At worst, the intervention is neutral."

His one concern, though—one that has been expressed by other researchers as well—is that some people may experience an uptick in LDL, the harmful form of cholesterol, even as their other markers improve. "This may be because some people interpret 'keto' as meaning they should eat as much butter and saturated fat as they can," Weiss says. "I don't think that means people have to come off keto—but they may want to reduce their intake of saturated fats, and replace those with mono- and polyunsaturated fats, while still keeping carbs very low."

Abdomen

Abdominal or "belly" fat has emerged as a major risk factor for many conditions, including heart disease, cancer and diabetes, because it can wrap around many of the surrounding organs and release toxins into them. The keto diet appears to be particularly adept at targeting this dangerous fat. A study in the *Journal of Nutrition* compared people on low-fat versus low-carb diets and found that the lower-carb dieters lost more "intra-abdominal adipose tissue."

In addition, a recent report from the NIH found that keto reduces weight,

"especially truncal obesity and insulin resistance." Message: Keto really helps whittle that waist!

Blood Sugar

Some of the strongest evidence of keto's benefits involves its effects on blood sugar—and by extension, on insulin resistance and type 2 diabetes. Insulin resistance happens when your body gets "worn out" by insulin spikes on a high-carb diet and stops responding as well to it, which can lead to diabetes (chronic high blood sugar). When you drastically limit carb intake, your pancreas doesn't need to pump out as much insulin, and your blood sugar levels stabilize. A study in the journal *JMIR Diabetes* showed that when people with type 2 diabetes followed a ketogenic diet for 10 weeks, not only did their blood glucose levels improve, but 57 percent of them were able to reduce or eliminate at least one diabetes medication. Other research shows similar results, including meta-analyses that evaluate many studies in order to see where the majority of the evidence points.

Even if you don't have type 2 diabetes, many people in the United States—an estimated one-third of the population—have metabolic syndrome, a precursor to diabetes and heart disease. The American Heart Association defines the syndrome as a cluster of risk factors, including abdominal obesity, high triglycerides, low HDL (good) cholesterol, high blood pressure, and high blood glucose. All of these risk factors have been shown to improve with a ketogenic diet. A study in *Diabetes India* followed people with metabolic syndrome who were put on one of three regimens: a keto diet, a standard American diet (typically high-carb), and a standard American diet plus exercise. The keto dieters showed greater

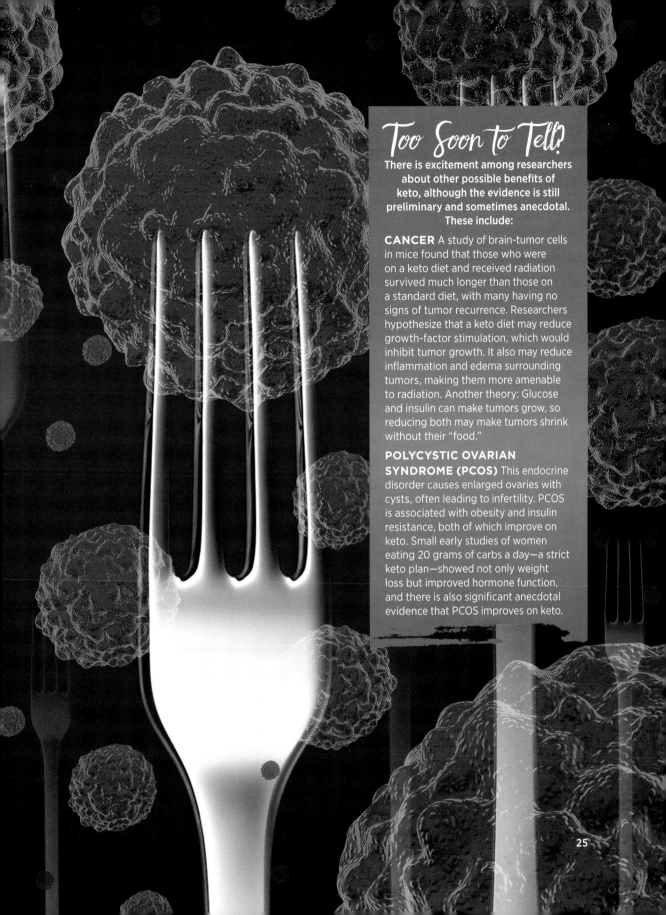

Too Soon to Tell?

There is excitement among researchers about other possible benefits of keto, although the evidence is still preliminary and sometimes anecdotal. These include:

CANCER A study of brain-tumor cells in mice found that those who were on a keto diet and received radiation survived much longer than those on a standard diet, with many having no signs of tumor recurrence. Researchers hypothesize that a keto diet may reduce growth-factor stimulation, which would inhibit tumor growth. It also may reduce inflammation and edema surrounding tumors, making them more amenable to radiation. Another theory: Glucose and insulin can make tumors grow, so reducing both may make tumors shrink without their "food."

POLYCYSTIC OVARIAN SYNDROME (PCOS) This endocrine disorder causes enlarged ovaries with cysts, often leading to infertility. PCOS is associated with obesity and insulin resistance, both of which improve on keto. Small early studies of women eating 20 grams of carbs a day—a strict keto plan—showed not only weight loss but improved hormone function, and there is also significant anecdotal evidence that PCOS improves on keto.

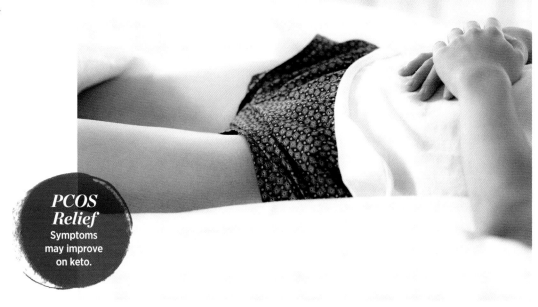

PCOS Relief Symptoms may improve on keto.

improvement than the others in weight loss, body-fat percentage, blood glucose levels, triglycerides and resting metabolic rate.

Metabolism

To many, one of the most frustrating elements of dieting is the fact that when you lose weight, your metabolism tends to slow down—requiring that the dieter eat less and less food to keep losing pounds, or even just to maintain the weight loss. Many experts feel it is this negative change in metabolism, rather than a failure of willpower, that makes the vast majority of dieters ultimately regain the pounds. But remarkably, keto diets don't appear to cause the same metabolic dip, and recent research shows that ketosis may even act to speed up the metabolism.

For a five-month-long clinical study in the journal *BMJ,* researchers compared dieters in three different groups—high-, moderate- and low-carb—while keeping their body weight stable so they could evaluate metabolic changes. "By preventing weight change, we could see how their metabolism changed as a direct response to dietary composition," explains the study's lead author David Ludwig, M.D., professor of nutrition at Harvard's T.H. Chan School of Public Health. And it turned out their metabolism differed remarkably, says Ludwig: "Total energy expenditure was about 250 calories a day greater on the low-carbohydrate diet compared to the high-carbohydrate diet." If researchers hadn't been working to carefully calibrate meals to keep weight steady, he adds, "this increase in metabolism would produce substantial weight loss. The study showed that the type of calories consumed affect the number of calories burned, challenging the long-standing dogma that all calories are alike to the body."

These results suggest why so many people manage to maintain their keto-based weight loss over time. The bottom line is that keto appears to make your body's "furnace" burn faster and hotter, boosting weight loss without forcing you to go hungry. That may end up being the definition of a "good diet."

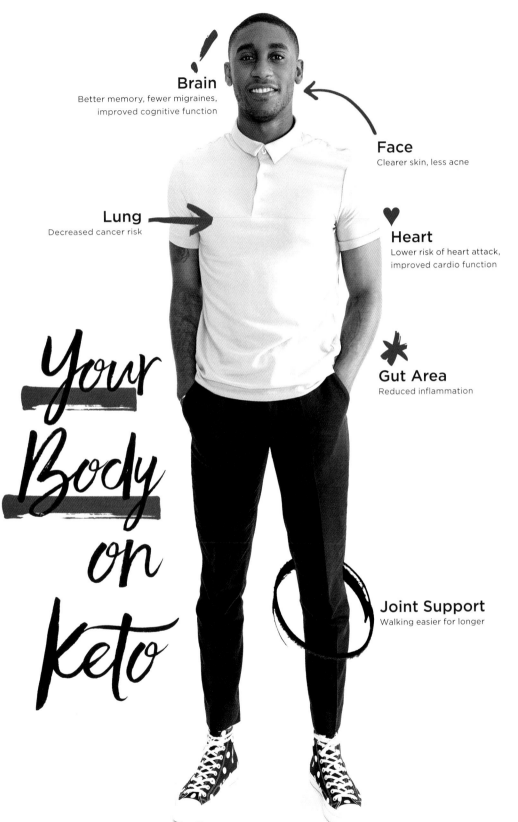

Brain
Better memory, fewer migraines,
improved cognitive function

Face
Clearer skin, less acne

Lung
Decreased cancer risk

Heart
Lower risk of heart attack,
improved cardio function

Gut Area
Reduced inflammation

Your Body on Keto

Joint Support
Walking easier for longer

Fats VS.

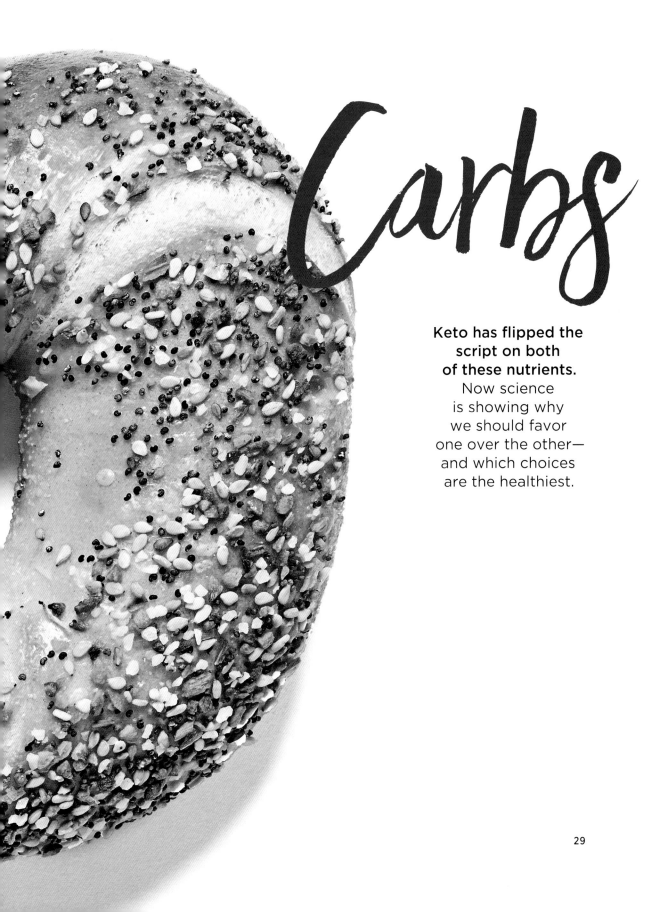

Carbs

Keto has flipped the script on both of these nutrients. Now science is showing why we should favor one over the other— and which choices are the healthiest.

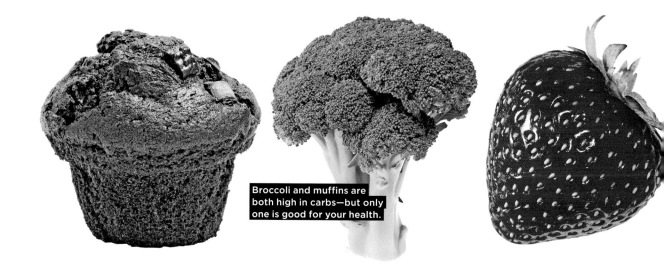

Broccoli and muffins are both high in carbs—but only one is good for your health.

The low-fat movement in the United States is so long-running—begun in the 1970s by dietary guidelines issued by the American Heart Association, and later adopted by the U.S. Department of Agriculture—that many people are still shocked when they hear how much fat they can eat on keto. For decades, we've been taught that "low fat" means "healthy," and that high-fat diets lead to obesity, heart disease and cancer. But science doesn't play favorites, and loads of research has increasingly shown that we should be eating drastically fewer carbs, and considerably more fat, while keeping protein intake moderate.

Many experts now feel that the obesity epidemic of the past few decades, as well as the meteoric rise in cases of type 2 diabetes, may in fact be a consequence of the low-fat trend. If you bring fat intake down, carbs will rise (there's only so much protein anyone can eat). Food manufacturers jumped on the low-fat bandwagon and started creating processed foods that replaced fats with carbohydrates, driving carb intake to new highs. The result: insulin resistance, diabetes and weight gain. "It's possible to think of the low-fat, near-vegetarian diet of the past half-century as an uncontrolled experiment on the entire American population," says Nina Teicholz, author of *The Big Fat Surprise*. "In 1961, roughly one in seven adult Americans was obese," she points out. "Forty years later, that number was one in three."

Once you understand how these two macronutrients work in the body, those stats are a lot less surprising. Here is what

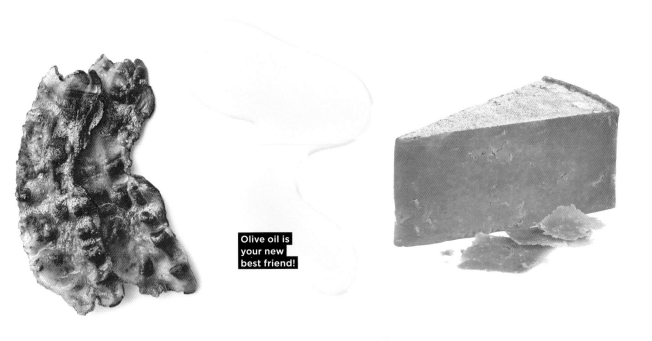

Olive oil is your new best friend!

researchers now know about the role of fats and carbohydrates, and how they affect your health.

The Return of Fats

Everyone remembers the days of low-fat margarines, nonfat sour cream, and reduced-fat cheeses and peanut butter; in fact, many of those products are still on shelves. Meanwhile, though, science has been overturning the low-fat apple cart. A large study in *Lancet* in 2015 summarized all major low-fat weight-loss trials and found no evidence that eating low-fat helps people lose weight, compared to any other diet.

At the same time, more research is showing that the opposite premise is true: that low-carbohydrate, high-fat regimens are more effective. Three large meta-analyses, which look at evidence from many studies, all in respected and peer-reviewed journals, found that low-carb diets consistently conveyed more benefits than low-fat. A 2015 study in *PLOS ONE,* after noting that a "low-fat diet is currently the recommended diet for overweight and obese adults," showed that low-carb diets outpaced low-fat plans both in weight loss and in cardiovascular health gains. The definition of "low-carb" in these studies was less than 120 grams of carbs a day, while strict keto calls for only 20 grams—so the benefits of keto could be even more powerful.

Which Fats?

Once you've decided to try a high-fat keto plan, that's the next question—and it's another area with controversy. In the decades when fat in general was decried as a health danger, one form of it was considered

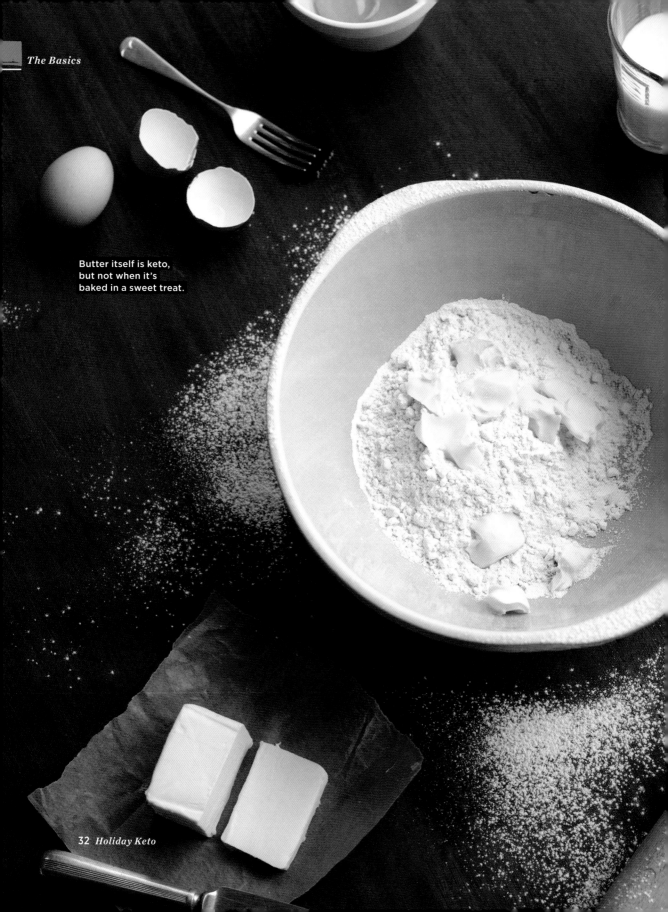

Butter itself is keto, but not when it's baked in a sweet treat.

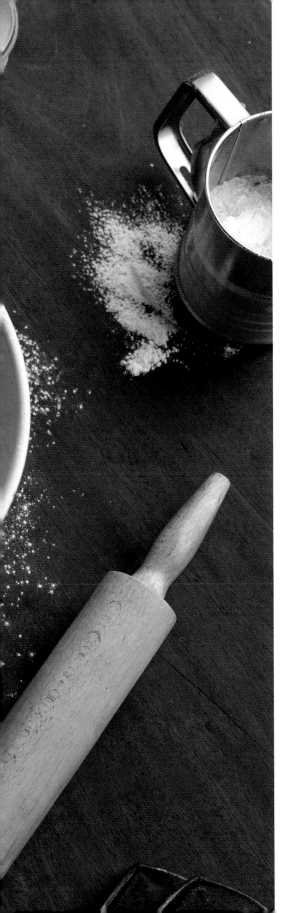

the greatest evil: saturated fat, which is derived mainly from animal sources and is solid at room temperature, like butter and lard. But research, again, is painting a different picture.

In the past decade, numerous studies have found no clear evidence of a causal link between saturated fat in the diet and heart disease, and therefore no reason to lower intake of it to under 6 percent, as the American Heart Association suggests. That's not to say that saturated fat is superior, experts add, but that it is likely a neutral in terms of health. Based on the recent evidence, a group of researchers suggested in an article in *The BMJ* in 2019 that the current recommendations by the World Health Organization to reduce saturated fat "fail to take into account considerable evidence that the health effects of saturated fat varies, depending on the specific fatty acid and on the specific food source."

If you are getting saturated fat from whole-food sources like eggs, dairy and grass-fed beef, alongside healthy fats like olive oil and omega-3s from fatty fish, you should be fine, says Kendra Whitmire, a functional nutritionist based in Laguna Beach, California. "Saturated fat got such a bad reputation because most studies were observational, and there were so many confounding variables, things like people smoking, or not exercising," Whitmire explains. "Then when further clinical studies came out, they showed that saturated fat is not really a strong factor." Even the Academy of Nutrition and Dietetics is now urging the USDA, in its next edition of nutritional guidelines for Americans, to "de-emphasize saturated fat as a nutrient of concern." In

Baker's Delight
You can still make holiday treats that are keto-friendly.

fact, the Academy explicitly stated in its letter to the USDA: "carbohydrate intake conveys a greater amount of cardiovascular disease risk than does saturated fat."

Unsaturated fats, on the other hand, have long been seen as healthy. These include fats in olives, avocados and many nuts, as well as omega-3 fatty acids (in fish, flaxseed and chia seeds). These are good for your heart, anti-inflammatory and possibly protective against cancer and neurodegenerative concerns like Alzheimer's disease.

The Fall of Carbs

Meanwhile, the carbohydrates that once dominated the base of the USDA food pyramid—grains, breads, cereals, rice, pasta— are now on many people's "out" list. How did they go from being lauded to avoided? It's a mirror image of saturated fats: Carbs were long seen as benign sources of calories, with the added benefit (at least with whole grains) of containing fiber. The low-fat movement pushed carbs into greater prominence, and many people felt that eating a bagel was healthier than eating steak. Then researchers dove deeper into the distinctions between highly processed carb foods (white bread, sugary cereals, sweets) and whole-food forms of carbs (fruits and vegetables are mostly carb, though many people don't realize that).

What studies found was that processed carbs break down very quickly in the body, causing a blood sugar spike followed by an insulin spike. Insulin is efficient at storing calories as fat, so many sweets end up going straight into storage. Then you're hungry all over again, setting up a boomerang effect— plus, you're gaining weight. Complex carbs from whole foods like broccoli or asparagus,

Good Carbs

Not all carbs are equal—high-fiber ones can help your gut.

on the other hand, not only offer many more nutrients for your body to use than a starchy carb item, but their fiber ensures that they break down slowly. They also simply contain fewer grams of carbohydrates—and much less sugar—so insulin doesn't have to come flooding in to lower blood sugar levels.

Choosing Your Carbs

The top-line message of keto is to realign your body's energy systems by greatly reducing carb intake—down to at most 10 percent, if not 5 percent, of calories. But the secondary message is more subtle: Not all carbs are bad, and you benefit from the nutrients in produce like cabbage and lettuce. The trick is both cutting carbs and being discriminating about those you *do* eat.

One easy way to choose carbs, says Andreas Eenfeldt, M.D., founder of Diet Doctor, is to look at where they grow. "Vegetables that grow above ground—things like lettuces, asparagus, cucumber, cauliflower, spinach and eggplant—tend to be lower in carbs and are best for keto," says Eenfeldt. "Below-ground vegetables, like white and sweet potatoes, beets, carrots and parsnips, are higher in carbs and should be avoided on a keto diet." For example, 100 grams of asparagus have 2 net carbs, while 100 grams of sweet potato have 17 grams, almost the daily total you're allowed on a strict keto plan.

The great thing about above-ground vegetables is that you can eat them almost without even counting, Eenfeldt adds. "It's hard to overeat spinach, zucchini, lettuce, asparagus and kale on a keto diet," he says. "Have them with butter or other sauces!" Then add salmon or lamb chops and you have a perfect keto dinner.

Winners

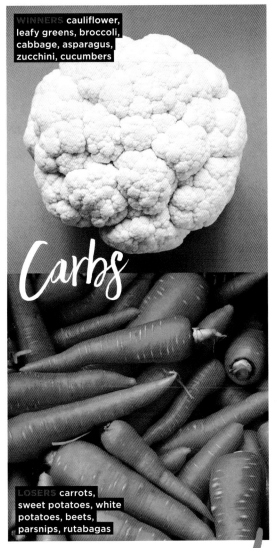

WINNERS cauliflower, leafy greens, broccoli, cabbage, asparagus, zucchini, cucumbers

Carbs

LOSERS carrots, sweet potatoes, white potatoes, beets, parsnips, rutabagas

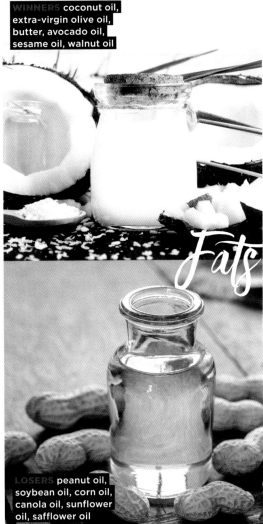

WINNERS coconut oil, extra-virgin olive oil, butter, avocado oil, sesame oil, walnut oil

Fats

LOSERS peanut oil, soybean oil, corn oil, canola oil, sunflower oil, safflower oil

AND Losers

Best Oils

These savory staples can help keep you in ketosis. Whether you prefer smoky, mild or nutty, the oils listed here provide health benefits along with flavor.

N ot all oils are created equal when it comes to the keto diet. Still, the monounsaturated and polyunsaturated fats found in natural oils contribute to keto's benefits, such as weight loss, a reduction in belly fat, and lower blood pressure. Here, we run down the very best keto choices.

Avocado Oil

Available as refined and unrefined, avocado oil—like the fruit itself—is full of healthy monounsaturated fat and oleic acid, which has been shown to help lower cholesterol. Also like the fruit, avocado oil has a creamy, rich (yet mild), almost buttery flavor, which makes it an ideal partner for cooking, as it doesn't interfere with the flavors of other ingredients. It has a very high smoke point and is ideal for roasting, grilling or sautéing veggies. It's also a good choice for salad dressings, pesto or dishes that use a variety of herbs.

Coconut Oil

Coconut oil is full of healthy saturated fats and lauric acid, both of which are thought to be easily converted to ketones and help to sustain ketosis. Its health benefits include helping to balance cholesterol and boosting metabolism. Relatively mild in flavor, it offers just a hint of its coconut roots—not the stronger taste of the dried coconut found in baked goods. It's suitable for both cooking and baking. Or add a scoop to a smoothie or even a cup of coffee. Coconut oil can be stored for a lengthy period of time without spoiling.

Macadamia Nut Oil

Not your everyday oil, macadamia nut oil's light flavor makes it a good substitute for butter or vegetable oils. High in monounsaturated fats, it's excellent for high-heat cooking, such as sautéing, and it also works well for baking. It can keep on your shelf for up to two years.

Olive Oil

Rich in monounsaturated fat and oleic acid, olive oil is one of the most versatile and trusty oils available. Extra-virgin olive oil is cold-pressed and is bottled after the first pressing. It is unrefined, and contains more of the nutrients from the olives. It tends to be a bit darker in color, and even a bit more earthy in flavor. The less-common virgin olive oil is also unrefined, but the production standards are not as stringent and it doesn't tend to be as flavorful as extra-virgin. Olive oil is suitable for grilling, roasting and sautéing. Its relatively mild flavor also makes it a reliable choice for salad dressings and drizzles.

Sesame Oil

Often used for Asian-influenced dishes, sesame oil has a slightly nutty flavor. Toasted sesame oil is also nutty with a hint of smokiness. Sesame oil is extracted from sesame seeds and is available as refined or unrefined. It serves up a blend of monounsaturated and polyunsaturated fats and is rich in antioxidants. The unique flavor of unrefined sesame oil is best for salad dressings and drizzles. Refined sesame oil can be used for sautéing and cooking.

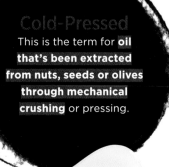

Cold-Pressed
This is the term for **oil that's been extracted from nuts, seeds or olives through mechanical crushing** or pressing.

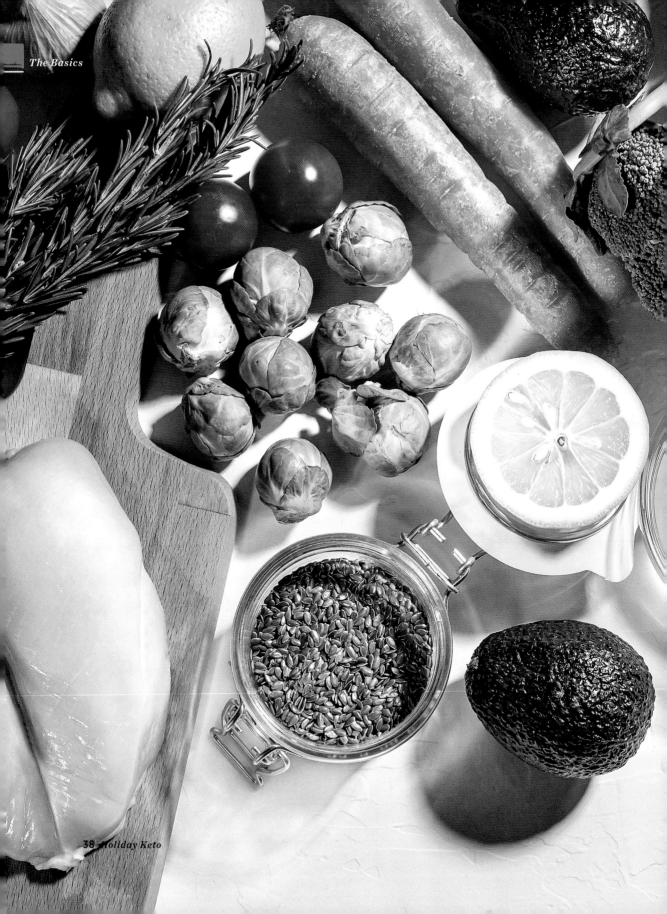

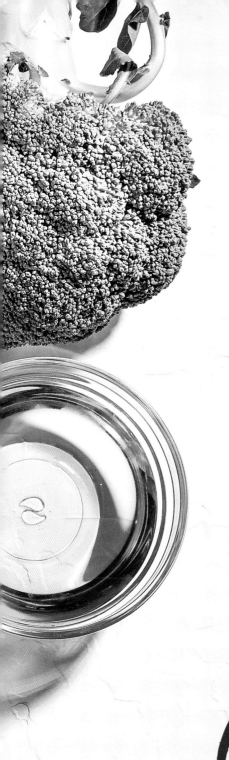

Keto
IN TERMS OF
Food

You know rice, pasta and potatoes
are off the table. **But what *can* you eat?**
A lot more than you may think!

f you're ready to put the keto diet into action, take a look at the different food categories—and what you can or can't eat from each. As you consider your macronutrient intake, it's important to think about the way in which you implement the diet. "Take two plates, for example: one of bacon, cheese and pork rinds, all keto foods that are high in fat and low in carbs; or one of what I'd recommend—a cut of high-quality animal protein, like good, fatty pork; a nonstarchy vegetable like broccoli; and some avocado, nuts and seeds. Focus on whole foods and don't forget fiber, micronutrients, vitamins and minerals," says wellness coach Tracey Grant, R.D.N.

Berries

Berries are low-ish in carbs and high in fiber, but you want to use them sparingly. Think of them more like a treat, says New York–based Kristen Mancinelli, R.D.N., author of *The Ketogenic Diet: A Scientifically Proven Approach to Fast, Healthy Weight Loss*. For example: Try sprinkling a few sliced strawberries on plain yogurt. And while blueberries are OK, blackberries, raspberries and strawberries have a higher fiber count, so are lower in net carbs.

Dairy and Eggs

Believe it or not, cheese is actually high in fat, protein and calcium but low in carbs. Finally, you can enjoy eating cheese and not worry about it! Cheese even contains conjugated linoleic acid, which has been linked to weight loss. Mancinelli notes that soft cheeses tend to have more grams of carbs, and hard cheeses have fewer. On the dairy front, plain Greek yogurt also fits the bill. Eggs are also OK: They are low (less than 1 gram) on the carb front, and one egg serves up just under 6 grams of protein.

Flours and Baking Ingredients

While still keeping an eye on your carbohydrate load, there are some flours

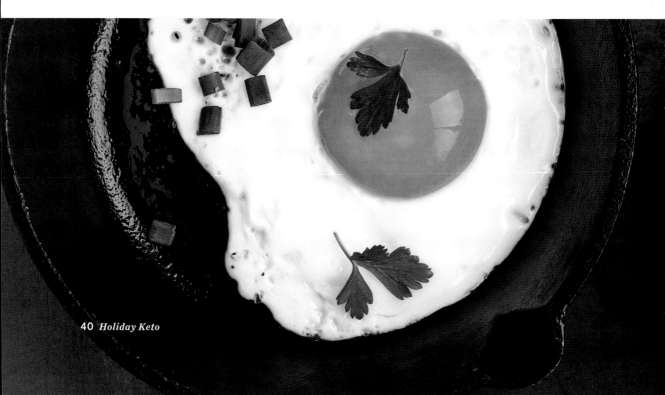

that are keto-friendly. These flours, not surprisingly, are derived from foods that are also keto-friendly, such as almonds and coconuts. If you need a binding agent to help these flours act more like wheat flour, xanthan gum will do the trick. And along these lines, salt, pepper and spices will help to enhance the flavor of any meal.

Nuts and Seeds

Nuts and seeds will be your friends on this diet, thanks to their healthy fat content as well as amino acids. They can also be rich in protein, vitamins, minerals, dietary fat and antioxidants. But be sure to focus on low-carb nuts. Cashews and pistachios, for instance, are higher in carbs.

Nut Butters

Nut butters not only taste good, but they also pack a protein punch. Try some on celery sticks or use them to make fat bombs. Keep nut butter single-serving pouches on hand—they're easy to eat while you're on the go. Just make sure they don't have added sugar; and try macadamia or pecan instead of peanut butter.

Proteins

Recommended proteins include low-carb seafood like salmon; shellfish are also usually low in carbs. Meat and poultry are staples of this diet; they contain no carbs but are rich in nutrients. "The flesh of animals other than shellfish does not contain carbohydrates; it's pretty much protein and fat," says Mancinelli. For the healthiest options, choose grass-fed or organic.

Veggies

Even veggies contain carbs. But when you look at the net carb count (subtracting the fiber from the carbs), you usually come up with a low-carb count with vegetables. The exceptions: starchy veggies, such as potatoes and butternut squash, which should be avoided. Focus on nonstarchy vegetables (see page 42 for low-carb veggie options).

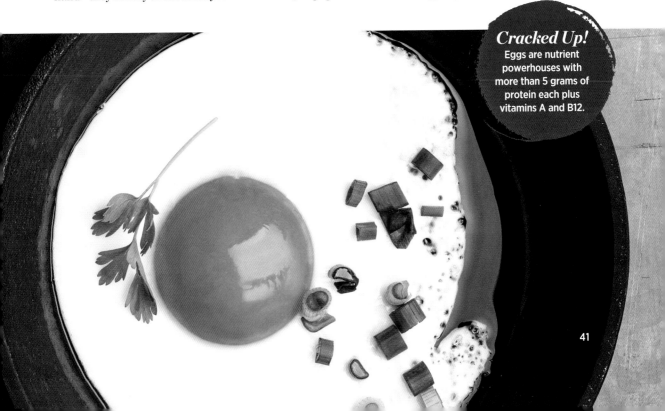

Cracked Up!
Eggs are nutrient powerhouses with more than 5 grams of protein each plus vitamins A and B12.

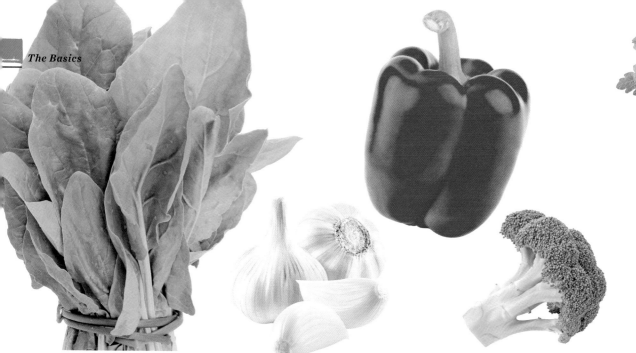

8 *Low-Carb* VEGGIES YOU

LEAFY GREENS

Lettuces, kale, chard and spinach, too: Leafy greens tend to be "all you can eat" foods. They are packed with nutrients, including vitamin K, and yet they are low in carbohydrates and have no-to-low impact on blood glucose. You can eat greens raw in a salad; place them in a blender to make a soup or smoothie; or sauté, bake or steam them to serve alongside a protein. Romaine lettuce can even be put on the grill.

GARLIC

By the numbers, garlic could be considered a high-carb food—1 clove of garlic contains 1 gram of carbs—but the amount that we typically eat at one time is so small that it counts as low carb. And we're thankful for that, because it packs a punch on the flavor front. Plus, numerous studies have shown that garlic may help to decrease blood pressure, boost the immune system and increase resistance to the common cold.

BELL PEPPERS

Choose from anti-oxidant rich red, yellow, orange or green peppers to snack on throughout the day, or mix them into a salsa or a salad. Fun fact: A pepper's carb content differs by its color. Green bell peppers have the lowest carb count, at 3 grams per 3.5 ounces; red has 4 grams and yellow has 5 grams. Of course, the brighter red and orange colors contain more carotenoids, which can offer more protective health benefits.

BROCCOLI

Like many of its fruit and veggie counterparts, broccoli (as well as other cruciferous vegetables, including cauliflower, Brussels sprouts and cabbage) is rich in antioxidants. These crunchy veggies contain active plant compounds called phytochemicals, which research has tied to protective health benefits. Broccoli has around 3 to 5 grams of carbs per 3.5 ounces. Try steaming, sautéing or roasting broccoli at 425°F.

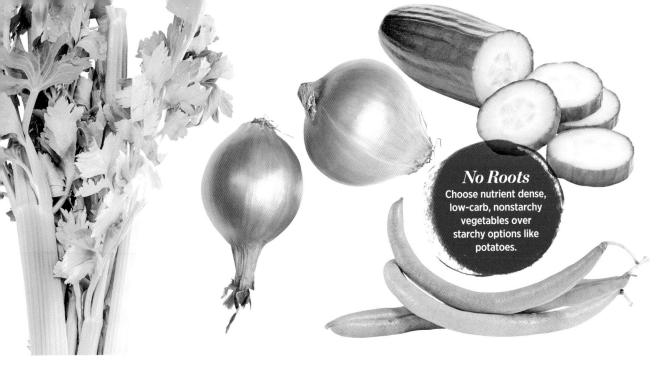

No Roots
Choose nutrient dense, low-carb, nonstarchy vegetables over starchy options like potatoes.

SHOULD KEEP IN YOUR FRIDGE

CELERY

Often thought of as the ultimate diet food, celery contains a mere 1 gram of carbs per 3.5 ounces. Despite it seeming like a watery, not-much-to-it veggie, celery is in fact an excellent source of fiber, and it's loaded with antioxidants, enzymes, vitamins and minerals. So cut it into sticks and keep it in the fridge for when you have a hankering for a crunchy snack, or chop it up and add to salads. Store celery in water to keep it fresh and prevent it from wilting.

ONION

Like garlic, onion is higher in carb content—7 grams per 3.5 ounces—yet it tends to be consumed in smaller amounts, which allows it to qualify as a low-carb veggie. **Onions are rich in fiber and the flavonoid quercetin, which also functions as an antioxidant.** Studies have tied quercetin to many health benefits, including lowering blood pressure. Try chopping up some onions to add to soups and salads.

GREEN BEANS

Although green beans are legumes, like lentils and chickpeas, they do not carry the same carb load that beans typically have. They have roughly 4 grams of carbs per 3.5 ounces. Green beans are a great source of fiber, and their rich green color is indicative of their chlorophyll content, which research has suggested may help protect against cancer. **Steam or sauté green beans in avocado oil; add them to a salad; or simply enjoy them raw as a snack.**

CUCUMBERS

At just 3 grams of carbs per 3.5 ounces, cucumbers are one of those snacks you could munch on all day. That's a good idea, considering they promote hydration, in addition to being rich in antioxidants. **Pair cucumber with all of its low-carb buddies— tomatoes, feta cheese, bell peppers, red onions and olives**—for a Mediterranean salad. For the dressing, combine olive oil, garlic and lemon juice with some salt and pepper to taste.

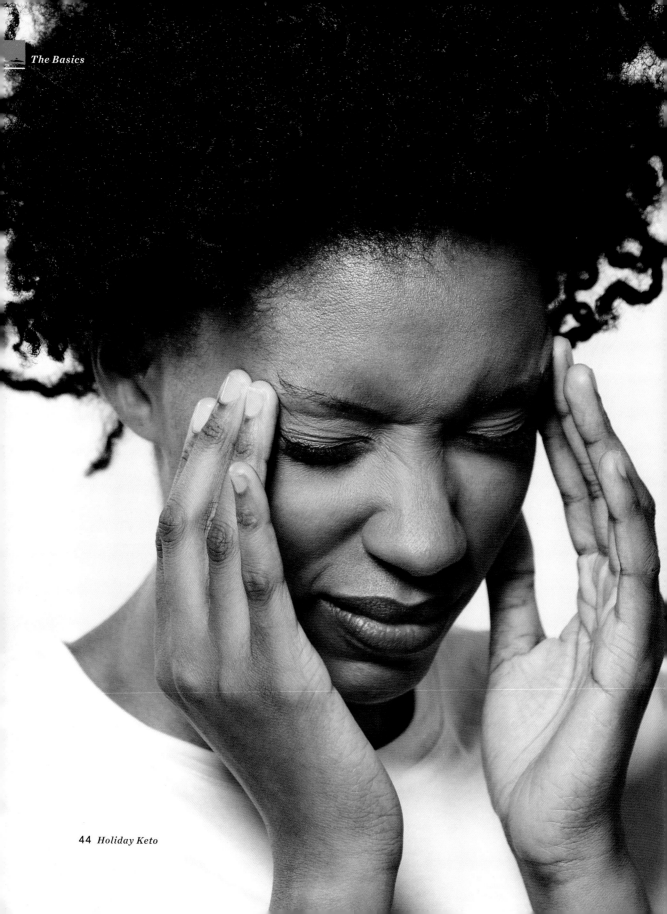

COPING WITH THE

Side Effects

There are plenty of positives the diet can provide, but—
especially in the early goings—there are also some downsides.
Banish them for good with these simple strategies.

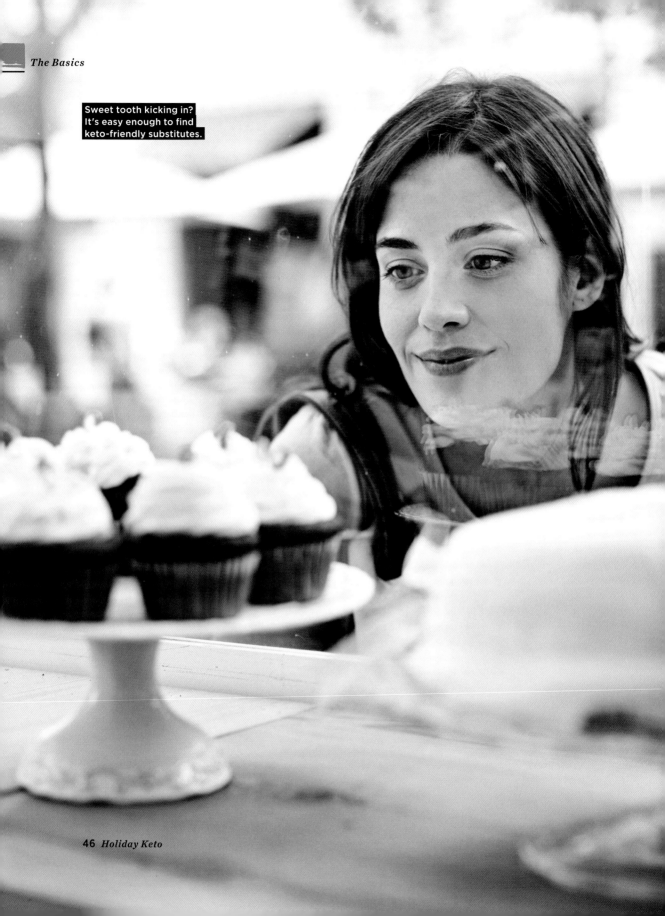

Sweet tooth kicking in? It's easy enough to find keto-friendly substitutes.

So you're psyched about going full keto. Your fridge is full of avocados, eggs and steak, and you've got the supplies for a year's worth of bulletproof-style coffee. Things are going great, you're already seeing results...then boom! Suddenly your head is throbbing with the keto flu, and your bad breath is rivaling the dog's.

Don't abandon ship at the first leg cramp! First of all, remember that these side effects are temporary and should abate as your body adjusts to its new role as a fat-burning furnace. Meanwhile, employ these tools to overcome the most troubling obstacles.

1 Keto Flu

You probably know by now that the keto flu isn't actually a flu at all; but that doesn't make the headaches, fatigue and mild nausea any more fun in the moment. And your friends and family probably aren't enjoying your brain fog much either.

THE FIX The good news is that most of the flulike symptoms aren't permanent. "Some report that the fog subsides after a few days; others report weeks," says Gabriele Geerts, R.D., a dietitian at Green Chef. "Think of it as caffeine withdrawal." You can generally avoid the flu funk altogether by upping your intake of water and salt. Most of the symptoms are caused by temporary dehydration and an increase in urine production as your body adjusts to the changes in diet. Drink a large glass of water with a spoonful of salt, and your troubles could be history within a half hour. If salty water doesn't appeal, try bone broth or bouillon.

2 Bad Breath

No one's favorite scent is nail polish remover, but that fruity bad-breath smell is actually from acetone, a ketone in your body. So if you've got that distinct smell on your exhales, congrats—you're doing the diet right and you've turned your body into a fat-fueled machine.

THE FIX If you don't like smelling like a nail salon, there are a few things you can do. First, maintain good oral hygiene by brushing your teeth twice a day. You can also use mouthwash and breath freshener to mask the odor—or you might want to try mints or gum (just be sure to pick sugar-free options). Nibbling on fresh mint leaves is a nice, natural antidote. Once again, make sure you're getting enough fluids, since dehydration doesn't help. And be patient—like most keto side effects, the bad breath tends to abate as your body adjusts.

3 Constipation

Not being able to go to the bathroom is never fun, but constipation can be an unfortunate side effect for those trying a low-carb diet for the first time, especially during the early weeks of adjustment.

THE FIX "With carbohydrates so limited, keto dieters often do not consume enough fiber," says Geerts. "Fiber stimulates the muscles of the intestines and keeps waste moving through the body; without fiber, the digestive process is slowed and less productive." While many fiber-rich veggies are no-nos for ketoers, low-starch vegetables, like cabbage and broccoli, can help. If you're still having trouble going No. 2, an occasional dose of milk of magnesia can get things moving again.

4 Leg Cramps

Leg cramps can certainly cramp your style during the first few weeks of a low-carb diet. And while they're usually minor, they can definitely derail your exercise program.

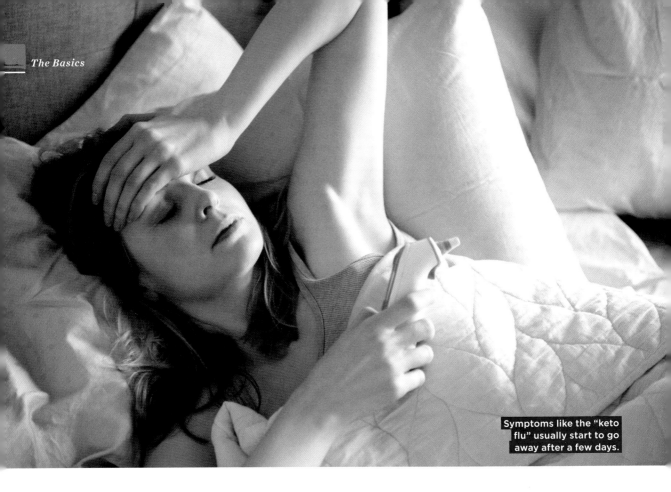

Symptoms like the "keto flu" usually start to go away after a few days.

THE AVERAGE AMERICAN EATS BETWEEN 225 AND 325 GRAMS OF CARBOHYDRATES PER DAY.

THE FIX Similar to keto flu symptoms, leg cramps are caused by a lack of minerals due to the increased urination. Once again, drinking water with a teaspoon of salt or sipping some broth can be an easy fix. If that doesn't work for you, try taking slow-release magnesium tablets to replace missing minerals. If all else fails, consider adding a few more carbs into the mix,

though obviously that can delay ketosis and weight loss.

5 Carb Cravings

You may not have realized how much you enjoyed snacking on chips at work or meeting pals for pizza and beer. Or maybe it's simply because you can't have something that you want it more.

THE FIX Geerts suggests giving pickles a go in place of crunchy carbs. "They're low in carbs but contain sodium and potassium to replenish electrolytes." Keto-friendly snacks, like pork rinds or Parmesan crisps, can also fill your need to munch. When cravings hit, it's also a good time to reach for a fat bomb, those keto specialities that ward off hunger pangs and boost fat macros.

Smart Swaps for Carb Lovers

Eating low-carb doesn't mean never tasting your favorite flavors.

When You Crave...

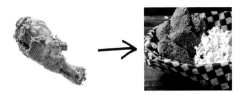

Fried Chicken If you've got a hankering for KFC, don't despair. You can still enjoy fried chicken—just use finely chopped pecans or pork rinds as the "breading" in place of bread crumbs.
SAVE 8 GRAMS CARBS

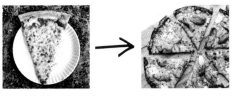

Pizza As the saying goes, even when pizza is bad, it's still pretty good, and it can still be good for your diet. Instead of using dough as the base, opt for cauliflower. You'll be amazed at how satisfyingly crispy this cruciferous vegetable substitute can be!
SAVE 21 GRAMS CARBS

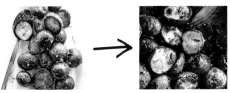

Roasted Potatoes Meat-and-potatoes meals can feel off-balance without the tubers. But radishes have the keto seal of approval, and roasting these root veggies makes them a wonderful substitute.
SAVE 19 GRAMS CARBS

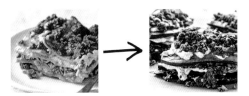

Lasagna Rich, savory lasagna is the perfect cure for a cold night, and ketoers are welcome to it—simply swap out the traditional pasta sheets for strips of thinly sliced zucchini or eggplant. Either is an ideal carb-free "pasta."
SAVE 20 GRAMS CARBS

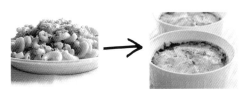

Mac and Cheese Mac and cheese might just be the king of all comfort foods, and you can still take comfort by using shirataki noodles instead of elbow macaroni. These "miracle" noodles are 97 percent water and have modest carbs, mainly in the form of glucomannan fiber.
SAVE 49 GRAMS CARBS

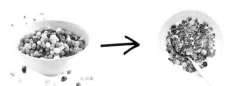

Cereal Mornings, for many people, mean a bowl of prepackaged cereal, like Frosted Flakes or Shredded Wheat. While those sugary, processed cereals won't fly on keto, you can enjoy a bowl of delicious coconut flakes and/or nuts-and-seeds cereals. There's even keto-friendly granola.
SAVE 12 GRAMS CARBS

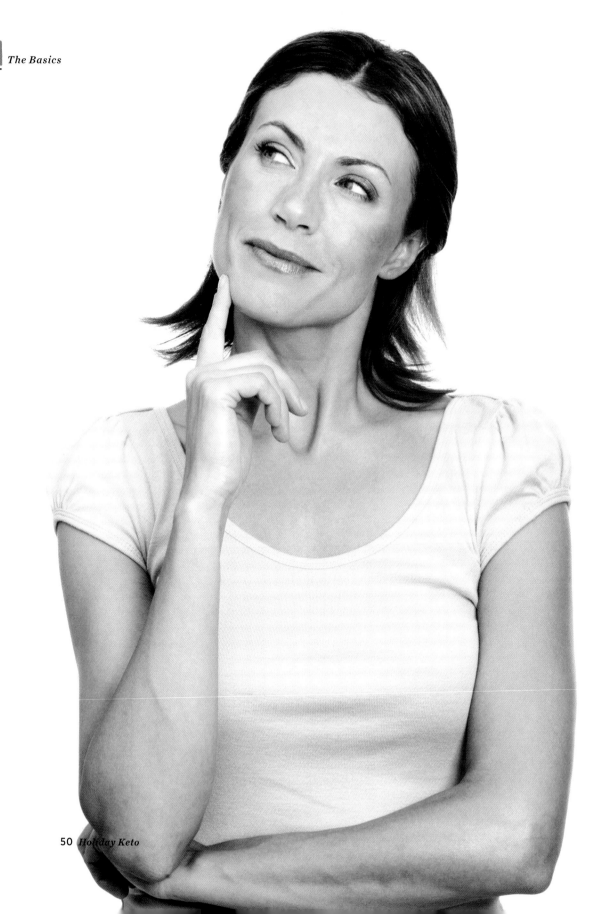

Glossary: KETO LINGO

Baffled by all the terms? Starting a new diet can be like trying to learn a new language. But here, we define the vocab you need to know to go keto.

BLOOD GLUCOSE Sugar found in the blood that comes from one's diet. The body readily burns glucose as energy, which is carried to the body's cells by the blood.

CARB CYCLING The process of systematically cycling periods of higher carbohydrate consumption into a low-carb diet. It's often associated with a performance-related goal.

CARBOHYDRATES A macronutrient, which when consumed becomes glucose, a primary source of energy for the body.

DIRTY KETO A keto diet that supports regular consumption of "dirty" or less healthy high-fat foods than are typically permitted when eating keto. This may include fast food and highly processed packaged foods.

ELECTROLYTES A mineral that has an electric charge in the body. Sodium, chloride, potassium and calcium are all types of electrolytes and can be found in such foods as dairy, nuts and salts. Electrolytes are essential for regulating fluid levels, supporting balanced pH levels and enabling muscle contractions.

EXOGENOUS KETONES Keto supplements designed to support the body in burning ketones as fuel rather than glucose. They are most commonly found sold as powdered ketone salts, which can be added to a liquid, or ketone esters sold as a liquid beverage.

GLUCOSE/GLYCOGEN A type of simple sugar and the primary source of energy in the body. It is formed when carbohydrates such as breads, fruits, vegetables and dairy products are broken down by the digestive system. Glucose is carried through the body by "blood glucose." Glucose that is not burned for energy is stored in the body as glycogen.

HDL CHOLESTEROL This "good" cholesterol scavenges "bad" LDL cholesterol and plaque from the arteries by sending buildup to the liver to be expelled by the body. Optimum levels of HDL (60 milligrams/deciliter and above) are associated with a reduced risk for heart disease, heart attack and stroke.

INSULIN A hormone produced by the pancreas, which allows glucose in the blood to enter the cells to be used as energy. Insulin prevents blood sugar levels from getting too high (hyperglycemia) or too low (hypoglycemia).

INULIN A type of fiber found in many plant foods that is not digested by the small intestine. As a supplement, inulin is often found in powdered form made from chicory

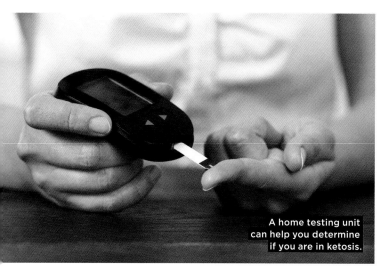

A home testing unit can help you determine if you are in ketosis.

root and consumed as a prebiotic. It can be taken to relieve constipation, for weight loss, to help control diabetes or simply for overall digestive health.

KETO FLU Symptoms such as headache, brain fog, fatigue and irritability that may occur two to seven days after beginning a keto diet. Keto flu is associated with the body's transition from burning glucose to ketones for fuel.

KETOGENIC DIET A low-carbohydrate, high-fat diet that puts the body in a metabolic state known as ketosis where it burns fat, rather than glucose, for energy.

KETONES A type of acid created from body fat produced by the liver to burn as fuel. The body creates ketones when it doesn't have sufficient glucose to fuel itself.

KETOSIS A metabolic state in which the body burns ketones rather than glucose for fuel. The ketogenic diet aims to induce ketosis for burning body fat.

INTERMITTENT FASTING Meal scheduling in which one does not eat, or severely reduces calories, for a determined period of time. Methods for intermittent fasting include: alternate-day fasting, periodic fasting, and time-restricted feeding, such as 14:10 (where you eat only during a 10-hour period each day, while fasting for the other 14 hours).

LDL CHOLESTEROL This "bad" cholesterol collects in the walls of blood vessels, where it can cause blockages. High LDL cholesterol (160 milligrams/deciliter and above) is associated with risk of heart disease, heart attack and stroke.

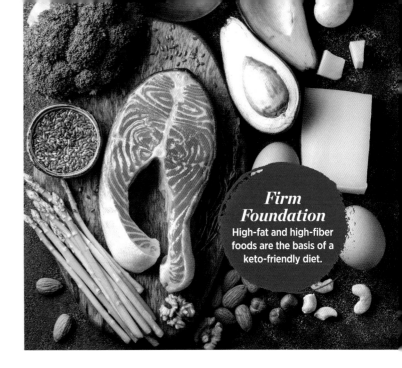

Firm Foundation
High-fat and high-fiber foods are the basis of a keto-friendly diet.

MACRONUTRIENTS (aka macros) A category of food required by the body in significant amounts. There are three macronutrients: carbohydrates (sugar), lipids (fat) and protein.

MCT OIL A supplement made of medium-chain triglycerides commonly extracted from coconut oil. MCT molecules are smaller than other fats, allowing them to enter the bloodstream more quickly and to therefore be more readily available for burning as fuel.

PREBIOTIC An indigestible fiber that feeds friendly bacteria in the gut and colon. Vegetables with high prebiotic content include chicory, Jerusalem artichokes and garlic.

TRIGLYCERIDES A type of lipid (fat) found in the blood. Triglycerides that are not used for energy are stored as fat. A high level of triglycerides in the blood can lead to pancreatitis, fatty liver, diabetes and heart attacks.

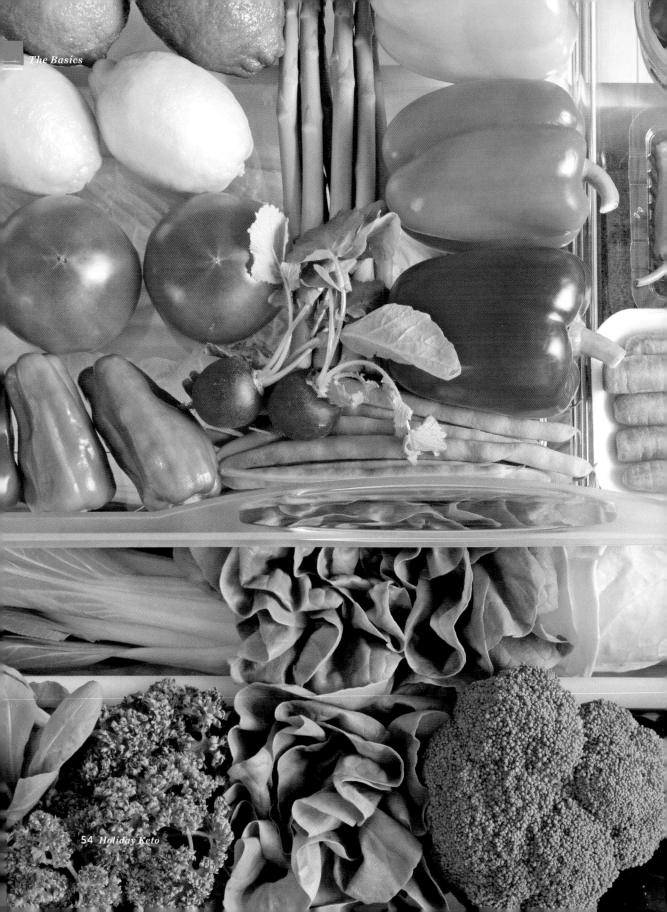

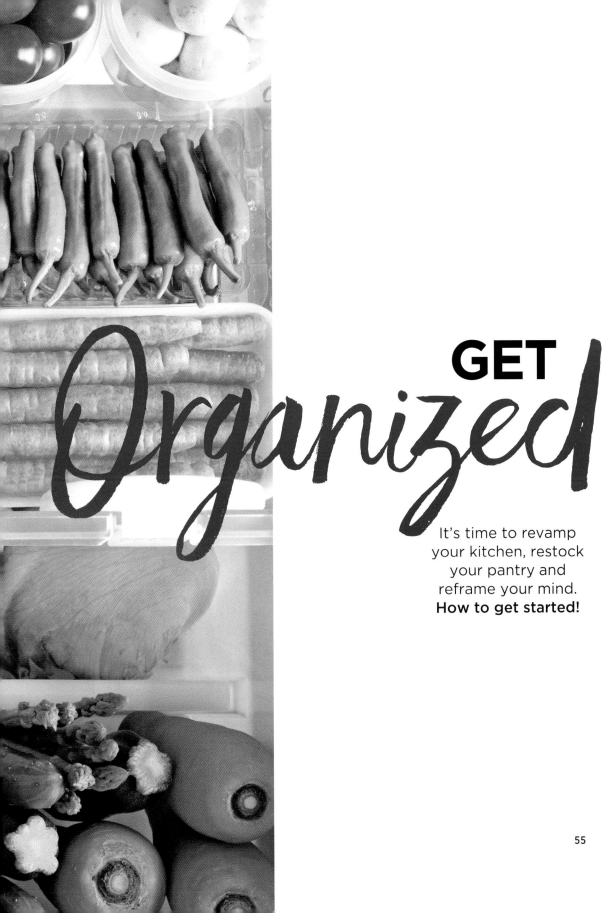

GET
Organized

It's time to revamp
your kitchen, restock
your pantry and
reframe your mind.
How to get started!

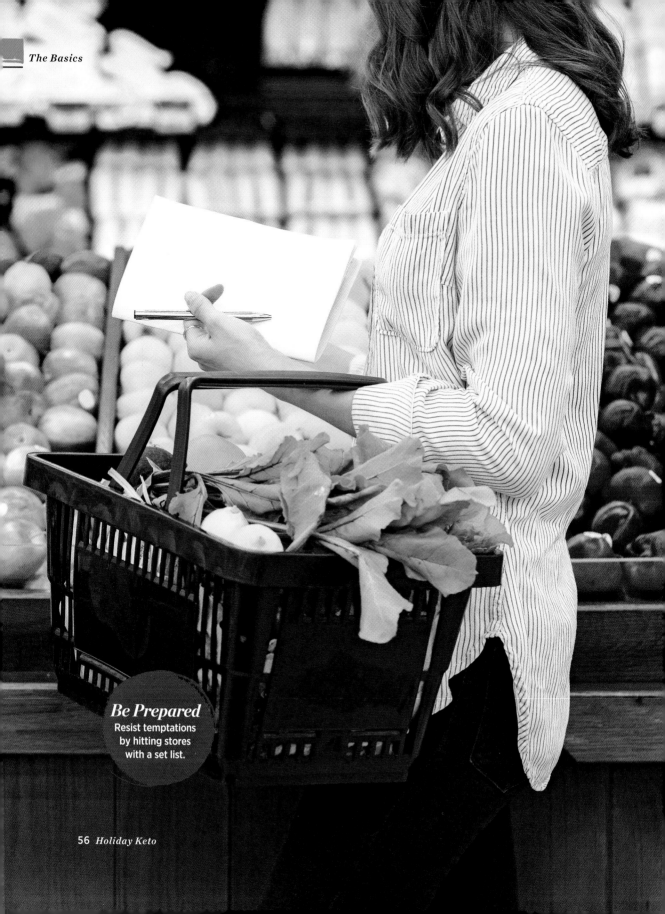

Be Prepared
Resist temptations by hitting stores with a set list.

"Give me six hours to chop down a tree, and I will spend the first four sharpening the axe," Abraham Lincoln once said. His sage mentality can also be applied to a ketogenic diet. Since eating low carbs and high fats contradicts many tenets of a standard Western diet, adopting the plan takes preparation and commitment. But laying the proper groundwork will help to ensure success down the road. Use this four-step strategy to transform your home from enemy territory to ground zero for keto success.

STEP 1
Clean Out

"Chances are you have a lot of kitchen go-tos that you'll need to toss," explains Anna Hunley, recipe developer and founder of Keto In Pearls (*ketoinpearls.com; @keto_in_pearls*). "You're going to be shocked when you realize all the unhealthy items you had lurking in your pantry." Why get rid of them altogether? Studies overwhelmingly support the idea that "out of sight, out of mind" has powerful benefits when it comes to diets. In other words, if you don't have cookies in the pantry, you're far less likely to eat them, explains Hunley.

STEP 2
Stock Up

"Your options are much more expansive when you cook your own keto food," says Hunley. "You can also monitor ingredients much more closely." All that at-home prep means keto cooks need all the help they can get. Among the most-prized kitchen devices: a spiralizer, which can transform vegetables such as zucchini into noodles (often called "zoodles") to use as a pasta substitute, and a food scale to measure meals down to the last macro. And, while most people already own a blender, you may want to consider upgrading to a heavy-duty food processor that can handle mincing thicker items like cauliflower and nuts.

STEP 3
Shop Smart

As you start shopping for healthier foods, you may find your trips to the grocery store take a new direction—specifically, around the outer edges. Grocers stock processed items, such as cereals and chips, in the central aisles, but many keto goodies—like meat, eggs and vegetables—are located on the perimeter of stores. Start prioritizing the outer edges and you'll be off to a good start when it comes to eating keto. (Though, Hunley reminds, you may want to do a quick trip down the middle for essentials like chicken stock and spices.)

STEP 4
Change Your Mind

While you whip your kitchen and pantry into tip-top keto shape, plan to get your brain in a healthier frame of mind, as well. "You wouldn't walk into a speech without preparing what to say first," says Hunley. "A diet is no different—you've got to get in the right mindset." As such, she recommends clearly defining for yourself why you are beginning keto. "Once you understand the why, it makes committing to the diet much more palatable." Another mental strategy: Add, don't subtract. Instead of focusing on the foods you're no longer eating, consider all the new delicious items you're adding to your daily lineup.

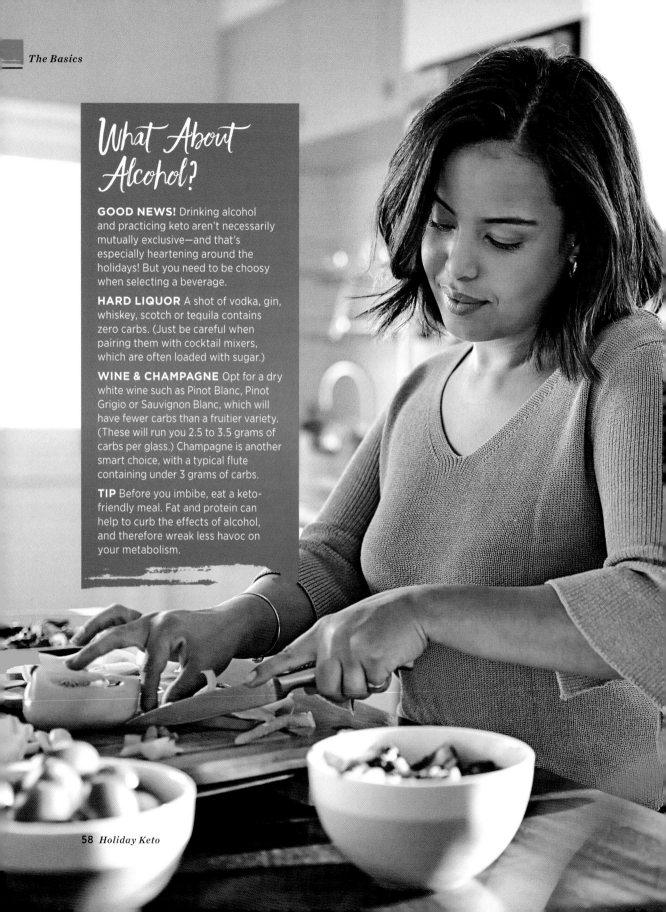

What About Alcohol?

GOOD NEWS! Drinking alcohol and practicing keto aren't necessarily mutually exclusive—and that's especially heartening around the holidays! But you need to be choosy when selecting a beverage.

HARD LIQUOR A shot of vodka, gin, whiskey, scotch or tequila contains zero carbs. (Just be careful when pairing them with cocktail mixers, which are often loaded with sugar.)

WINE & CHAMPAGNE Opt for a dry white wine such as Pinot Blanc, Pinot Grigio or Sauvignon Blanc, which will have fewer carbs than a fruitier variety. (These will run you 2.5 to 3.5 grams of carbs per glass.) Champagne is another smart choice, with a typical flute containing under 3 grams of carbs.

TIP Before you imbibe, eat a keto-friendly meal. Fat and protein can help to curb the effects of alcohol, and therefore wreak less havoc on your metabolism.

The Ultimate Keto Shopping List

Consider this your pantry primer for all things delicious and keto.

FATS & OILS
- [ ] Avocado Oil
- [ ] Butter (grass-fed)
- [ ] Coconut Butter
- [ ] Coconut Oil
- [ ] Extra-Virgin Olive Oil
- [ ] Flaxseed Oil
- [ ] Ghee
- [ ] MCT Oil
- [ ] Sesame Oil

POULTRY
- [ ] Chicken (with skin)
- [ ] Duck
- [ ] Turkey

MEAT
- [ ] Bacon (nitrate free)
- [ ] Bison
- [ ] Ground Beef
- [ ] Ham (no sugar)
- [ ] Lamb
- [ ] Pork Chops
- [ ] Pork Loin
- [ ] Sausage
- [ ] Steak (well marbled)
- [ ] Veal

SEAFOOD
- [ ] Anchovy, Mackerel and Sardine Fillets
- [ ] Canned Salmon and Tuna
- [ ] Fresh and Smoked Fish

MISCELLANEOUS
- [ ] Bone Broth
- [ ] Eggs

DAIRY
- [ ] Cheese (firm) (Cheddar, Colby, Jack, Parmesan, Swiss)
- [ ] Cottage Cheese
- [ ] Cream Cheese
- [ ] Feta
- [ ] Goat's Milk Cheese
- [ ] Heavy Cream
- [ ] Sour Cream
- [ ] Yogurt

FRUITS
- [ ] Avocados
- [ ] Blackberries
- [ ] Blueberries
- [ ] Lemons and Limes
- [ ] Olives
- [ ] Raspberries
- [ ] Strawberries

VEGETABLES
- [ ] Asparagus
- [ ] Bell Peppers
- [ ] Broccoli
- [ ] Brussels Sprouts
- [ ] Cabbage
- [ ] Cauliflower
- [ ] Celery
- [ ] Cucumbers
- [ ] Garlic
- [ ] Greens
- [ ] Kale
- [ ] Lettuce (all types)
- [ ] Mushrooms (all types)
- [ ] Onions
- [ ] Radishes
- [ ] Shallots
- [ ] Spaghetti Squash
- [ ] Spinach
- [ ] Tomatoes (fresh and canned whole)
- [ ] Zucchini

NUTS & SEEDS
- [ ] Almonds
- [ ] Almond Butter
- [ ] Almond Flour
- [ ] Brazil Nuts
- [ ] Cashews
- [ ] Chia Seeds
- [ ] Coconut Flakes
- [ ] Coconut Flour
- [ ] Flaxseeds
- [ ] Hemp Seeds
- [ ] Macadamia Nuts
- [ ] Pecans
- [ ] Pine Nuts
- [ ] Pistachios
- [ ] Pumpkin Seeds
- [ ] Sesame Seeds
- [ ] Sunflower Seeds
- [ ] Tahini
- [ ] Walnuts

CONDIMENTS & SEASONINGS
- [ ] Apple Cider Vinegar
- [ ] Balsamic Vinegar
- [ ] Cinnamon
- [ ] Coconut Aminos
- [ ] Dill Pickles
- [ ] Erythritol
- [ ] Hot Sauce
- [ ] Kimchi
- [ ] Monk Fruit Sweetener
- [ ] Mustard
- [ ] Salsa
- [ ] Sauerkraut
- [ ] Stevia
- [ ] Swerve
- [ ] Vanilla Extract
- [ ] White Vinegar

EXTRAS!
- [ ] Cacao Nibs (unsweetened)
- [ ] Cacao Powder
- [ ] Collagen Protein Powder
- [ ] Dark Chocolate
- [ ] Flaxseed Crackers
- [ ] Parmesan Crisps

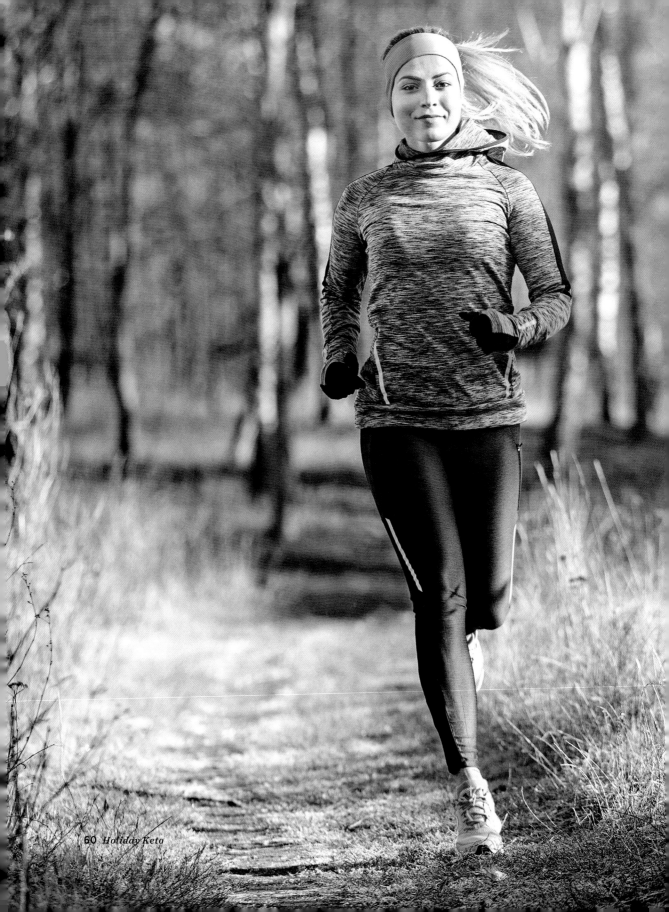

Chapter 2

Seasonal Strategies

HAVE A HAPPY, HEALTHY HOLIDAY WITH THESE TIPS.

Survive
THE SEASON

Thanksgiving feasts.
Holiday festivities.
New Year's libations.
Game-day dips.
**Keto practitioners
share ways to stay
strong amid timely
temptations.**

Cheers! You can still be
the life of the party when
following the keto diet.

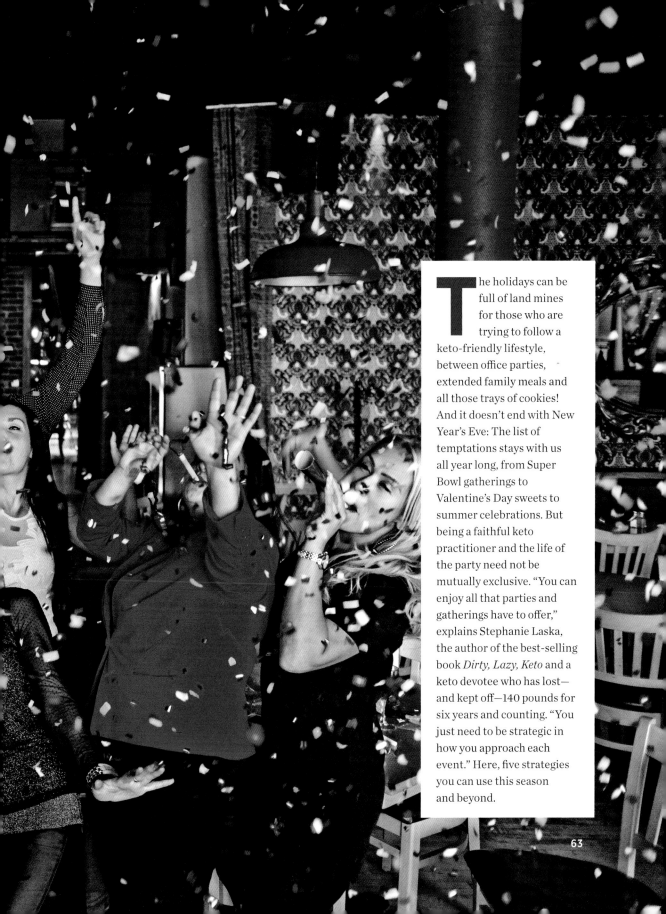

The holidays can be full of land mines for those who are trying to follow a keto-friendly lifestyle, between office parties, extended family meals and all those trays of cookies! And it doesn't end with New Year's Eve: The list of temptations stays with us all year long, from Super Bowl gatherings to Valentine's Day sweets to summer celebrations. But being a faithful keto practitioner and the life of the party need not be mutually exclusive. "You can enjoy all that parties and gatherings have to offer," explains Stephanie Laska, the author of the best-selling book *Dirty, Lazy, Keto* and a keto devotee who has lost—and kept off—140 pounds for six years and counting. "You just need to be strategic in how you approach each event." Here, five strategies you can use this season and beyond.

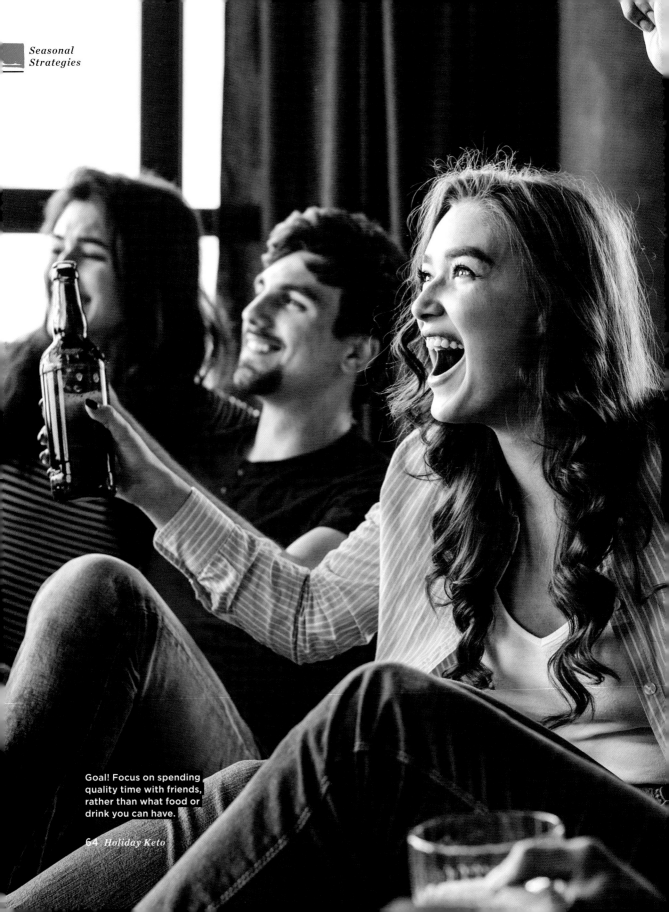

Goal! Focus on spending quality time with friends, rather than what food or drink you can have.

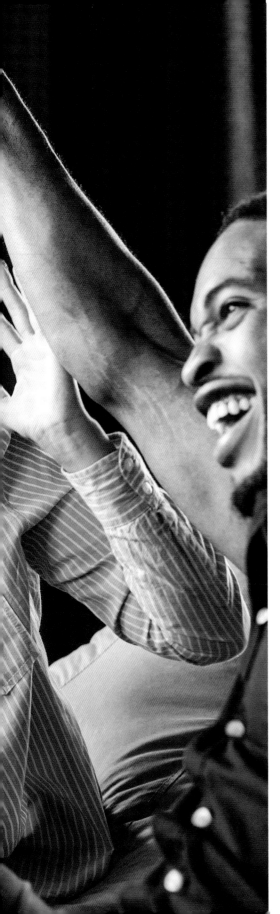

STRATEGY #1
Reframe the Occasion

"Holidays are really all about carrying on traditions. And for many people, those traditions center around food," says Laska. That connection, however, is largely misguided. Often simply identifying the underlying impetus for a tradition is enough motivation to incite change. "I found myself making my grandmother's (very unhealthy!) recipes for family gatherings," Laska recalls. "But then I expanded my notion of how to honor her. I came up with new ways to carry on her memory, like using her china." Suddenly, Laska's need to whip up carb-filled treats was gone.

The same cognitive switch can apply to any get-together, not just sentimental ones. Super Bowl parties, for example, aren't founded on celebrating the splendor of nachos—it's an opportunity to spend time with friends and take in a good game. When you go into an event with the intentions clearly framed, you'll have a far easier time skipping the unhealthy foods and focusing on all the fun.

STRATEGY #2
Shed the Shame

Dietary restrictions and sensitivities are now part of the national vocabulary. (Please take a moment and try to recall a restaurant menu that didn't mention "gluten-free" or "vegan" somewhere on it.) This commonality is great news for those of us making health-based lifestyle choices. "People with gluten intolerance or dairy sensitivities have been emboldened to make their needs known," says Alex Reed, editor in chief of the website Bodyketosis. That is to say, individualized eating approaches have become normalized and valued here in the United States. Why should it be any different for keto adherents? Reed encourages keto eaters, or those following any diet for that matter, to not feel shy about speaking up when it comes to their specific restrictions. "Your eating habits are based on a desire to obtain a healthier lifestyle and be the best you possible," Reed says. So how do you get the word out? A simple call to a host before a get-together can alleviate big headaches and temptations the day of the event. "Explain your constraints and mention items that are good for you, too, such as veggies and meats," Laska adds. "Most hosts want nothing more than their guests to feel included and well-fed!" Bonus: Making your eating habits known this go-round can only set you up for success at the next gathering, as well.

STRATEGY #3
Give to the Cause (Or the Host!)

While it's important to speak up about your eating habits, there's also no need to put pressure on the host. "I've gotten in the habit of asking each host what I can bring, even if it's not a potluck," explains Laska. "That way I know there will be at least one dish that's a slam dunk for me. And the host is almost always grateful for a little help." This is also an opportunity to introduce friends to the delicious dishes that come with keto. "You can surprise fellow partygoers big time," says Reed. "I bet they would have never guessed those bite-size keto pizzas or spicy chicken wings are a 'diet food.'"

To really take charge of your eating, host your own party. "There's no better way to stay on top of what you're consuming than to plan the menu yourself," Reed says.

Keep one or two non-keto items on the menu, but get creative and surprise guests with the wonders of keto eating. A girl's-night Valentine's gathering with chocolate fat bombs instead of run-of-the-mill chocolates? Sounds like a fun and indulgent occasion to us!

STRATEGY #4
Lean in to Your Habits

"Willpower will get you only so far," says Reed, who encourages keto eaters to have their habits fine-tuned before they dive into the party scene. You wouldn't try to ride a motorcycle down the interstate on your first try. The same idea of practice can be applied to keto. "You need to have made keto eating the norm before you surround yourself with carb-filled temptations," Reed adds.

Becoming familiar with your habits and tendencies will help you to make better decisions, explains Laska. "You may realize that you're golden in the mornings on through lunchtime, but in the evenings, when you're tired, you're more likely to slip," she says. "With that in mind, you'll know to be on better alert and more aware at a nighttime event."

One way to test your habits before a party? Do a trial run at a restaurant with a few friends. Practice ordering the good-for-you items off the menu. You'll be surprised how this helps make such decisions second nature when you're in the "wild" of a buffet-style party or near a box of candy, adds Laska.

STRATEGY #5
Embrace the Big Why

Both Laska and Reed remind us that it's imperative to hold fast to your reasons for beginning keto in the first place, whether

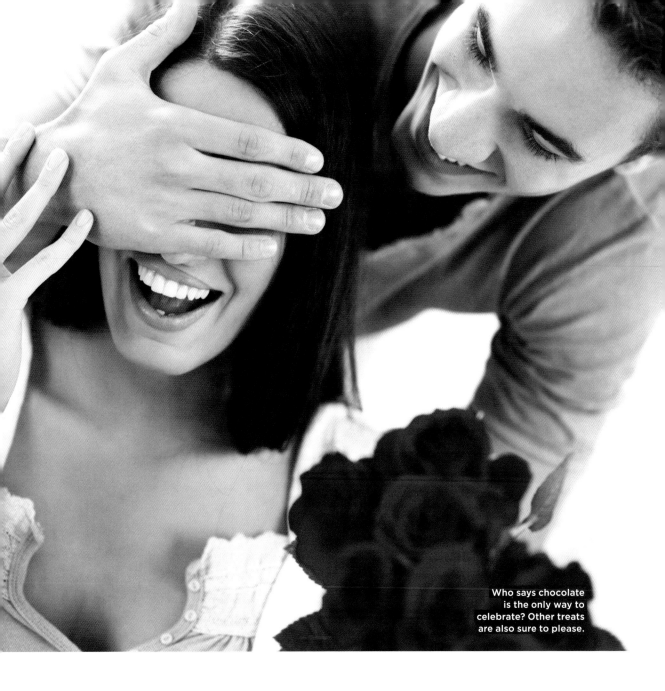

Who says chocolate is the only way to celebrate? Other treats are also sure to please.

that's weight loss, improved brain function or better management of a condition such as diabetes. "My motivation to eat well is to have the best health possible," says Laska. "Reminding myself of that aim truly helps to keep it all in perspective."

In fact, studies show that understanding and reminding yourself of those underlying values will go a long way in helping you stick to your goals. (Writing down your objectives and reviewing them before a party can also be beneficial.) As Reed points out, when you keep the big picture in mind, abstaining from that pink-frosted Valentine's Day donut in the office break room seems like a much smaller hurdle to overcome.

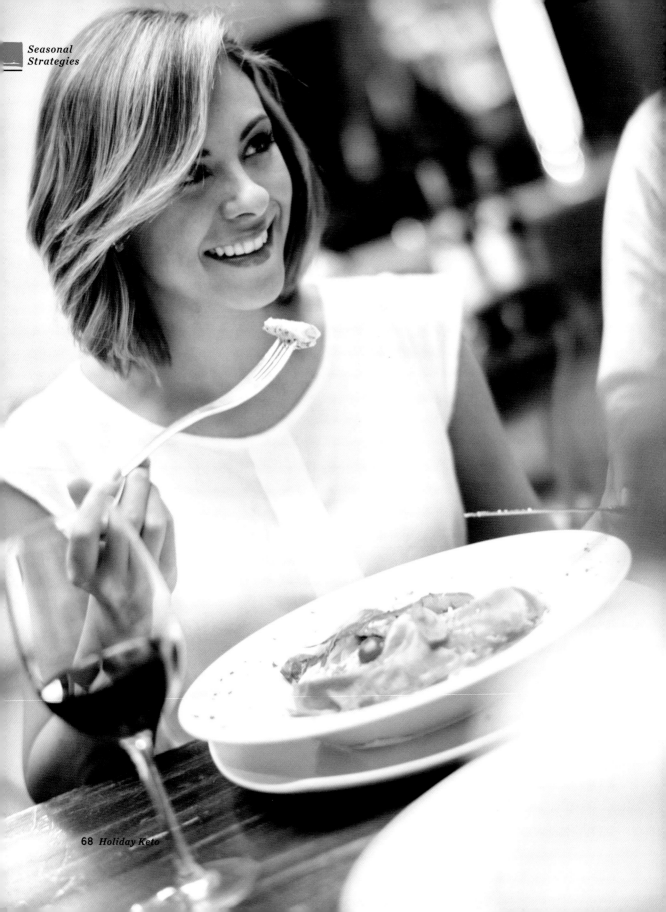

TABLE
FOR
One

Plan ahead during party season.
These tips will help you stick to
your diet through the holidays—
no matter how much everyone
else is indulging.

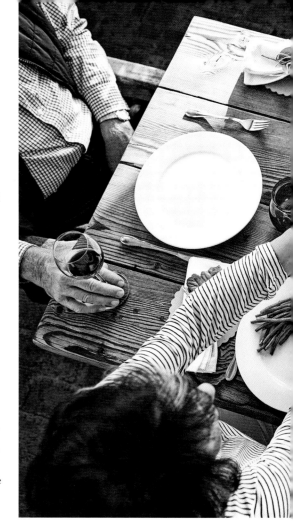

When you're facing a holiday whose very claim to fame is feasting (looking at you, Thanksgiving), people can take it a little...personally if you refuse to participate in an all-out binge. There could be any number of reasons: Your self-control could provoke food guilt in others. Aunt Mary may take it as a personal slight that you're not indulging in her famous cranberry-lattice pie. They may feel you're showboating, or genuinely worry that your keto adherence is a sign of a food pathology. Whatever prompts it, though, the pushback is awkward. Here's some expert advice on how to deflect—nicely.

What to Say...

...Aside from "mind your own business," of course. Your family and friends may actually be concerned about keto, which has received some skeptical press in places. "People you're eating with may be confused about the new dietary pattern you're following," says Ginger Hultin, M.S., R.D.N., a Seattle-based dietitian and spokesperson for the Academy of Nutrition and Dietetics. "You could say something like, 'I know you care about me, but I'm working with my doctor on this diet and it's prescribed, for a specific reason, for my health," advises Hultin. "Let them know all the healthy foods you can eat, like green veggies, fresh meat, seafood and poultry."

It also makes sense to alert your host beforehand about your way of eating, says keto coach Mandy Pagano. "If you stay quiet about it, don't be shocked when you show up to find a table full of nothing you can eat." Of course, it helps if in the same breath you offer to bring some wonderful keto-friendly side dish or dessert.

Pagano also stresses being prepared to stand up for yourself, politely but firmly.

"Ideally, everyone is going to be super-stoked for your keto progress and completely understanding about your new dietary needs, but realistically, that's not likely to happen," she says. "So you may receive pushback, or flat-out pushiness, regarding your food choices and any abstinence from holiday favorites." The key is to calmly assert yourself, and not let anyone "bully you into eating non-keto foods," says Pagano. If you do give in to pressure "just this time," you'll face it again next time, "so nip it in the bud."

What to Do

Number-one tip: Plan ahead. "You don't want to arrive hungry and then spend the

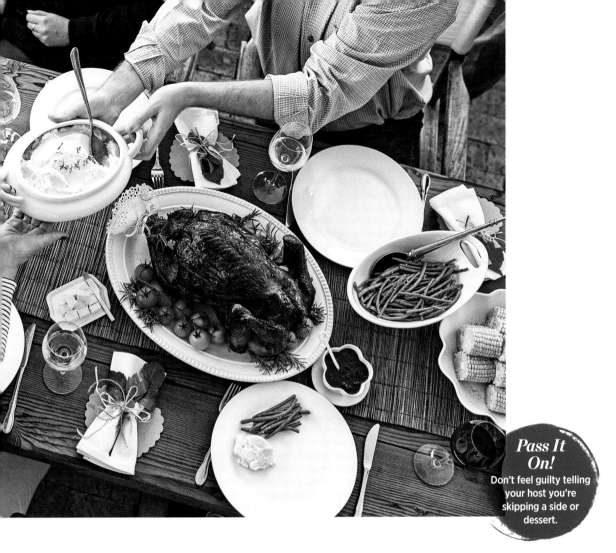

next two hours staring at crackers, chips and brownies," says Louise Hendon, co-founder of The Keto Summit and author of *The Essential Keto Cookbook*. Have a nice keto nosh before you go, so you won't have a growling stomach. You might also give yourself a little talking-to at the same time. "Before heading out of the house, mentally prepare yourself to stick to keto," says Hendon. "You've been to plenty of these parties before, so you know what foods to expect and what foods to avoid." Visualization is powerful.

Lastly, Pagano says, remember the reason for the season. "Thanksgiving is about being thankful for the blessings we have, and that includes spending time with our loved ones. Christmas and Hanukkah are about God and his gifts to us. If you celebrate a secular winter holiday, it's about family and loving your neighbor." Yes, sharing food, breaking bread together, is part of how we celebrate, but it's not everything. If you're focused on how you can't eat some carb-y side dish, you may be missing the point.

Above all, Hendon urges, "Don't stress too much! This is the season to be merry. If you want to stick 100 percent to keto during the holidays, plan ahead to do so. And if you want to let go a bit and eat pie on Christmas, just choose to do that, and then go back to keto the next day."

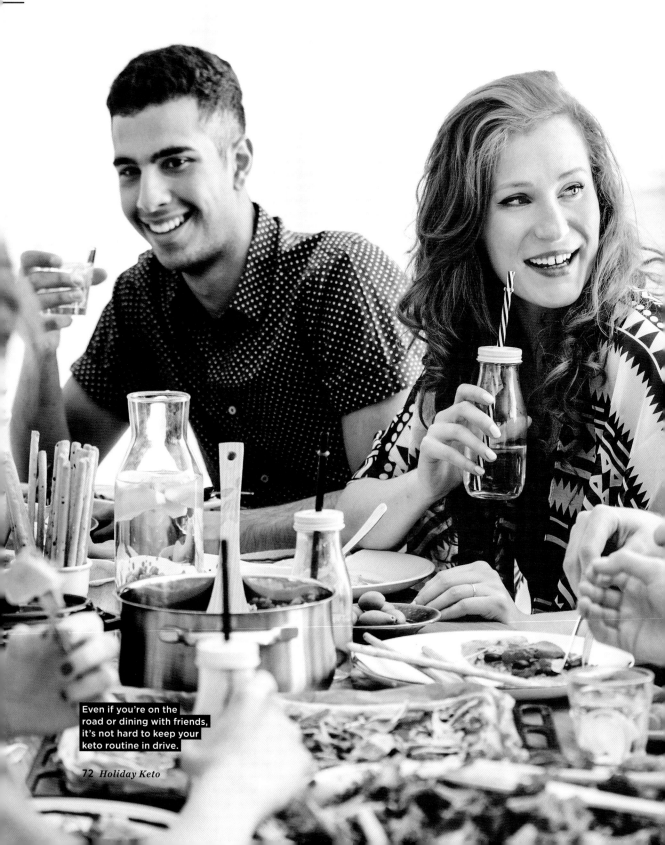

Even if you're on the road or dining with friends, it's not hard to keep your keto routine in drive.

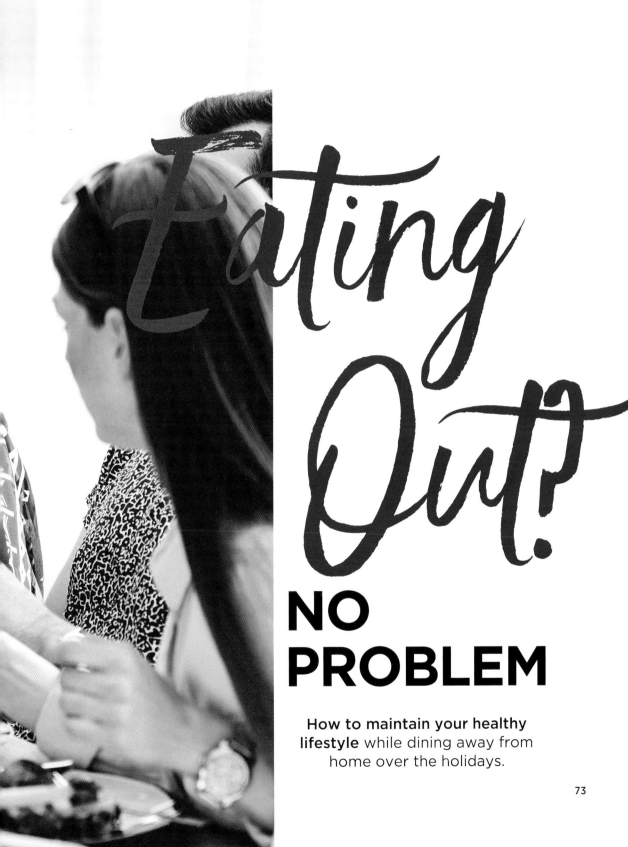

Eating Out?

NO
PROBLEM

How to maintain your healthy lifestyle while dining away from home over the holidays.

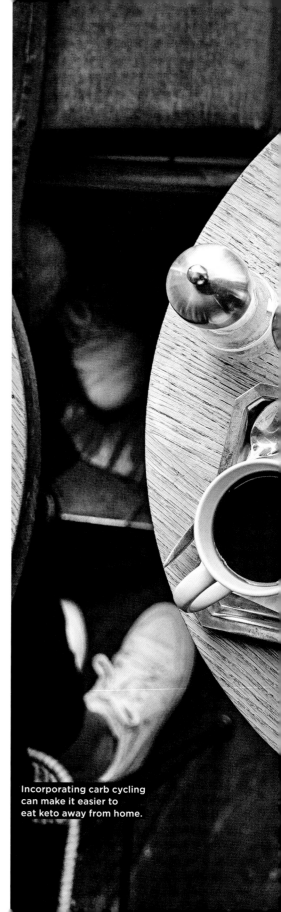

So, you've finally gotten the hang of this keto thing. You're no longer driven by cravings, the brain fog has cleared, and your pants are fitting better. Or perhaps you're not quite there, but you're committed to this way of eating, and your fridge and pantry are stocked with the requisite meats, nuts and snacks cultivated from careful label-reading and food prep. You're sailing along in your healthy food routine and then...fa, la, la, the holiday season comes roaring around the corner and you're headed off on vacation or to visit far-flung family. Can you keep your healthy habits when carb-laden foods fly your way with each passing mile? Is it possible to find keto-friendly foods on the go?

Success boils down to one thing, says Angela Mavridis, holistic nutritionist and CEO and founder of Los Angeles–based TRIBALÍ Foods, which specializes in keto, paleo and Whole30 snacks: "You have to plan. Those who don't plan, fail," she says. "When you're at home and you know

Be Nice to Yourself

If you do end up eating that Christmas cookie, don't beat yourself up. **"If it's a special thing, just make that your 'carb day,'" says holistic nutritionist Angela Mavridis.** "Feeding yourself healthfully while maintaining sanity is what's really important."

Incorporating carb cycling can make it easier to eat keto away from home.

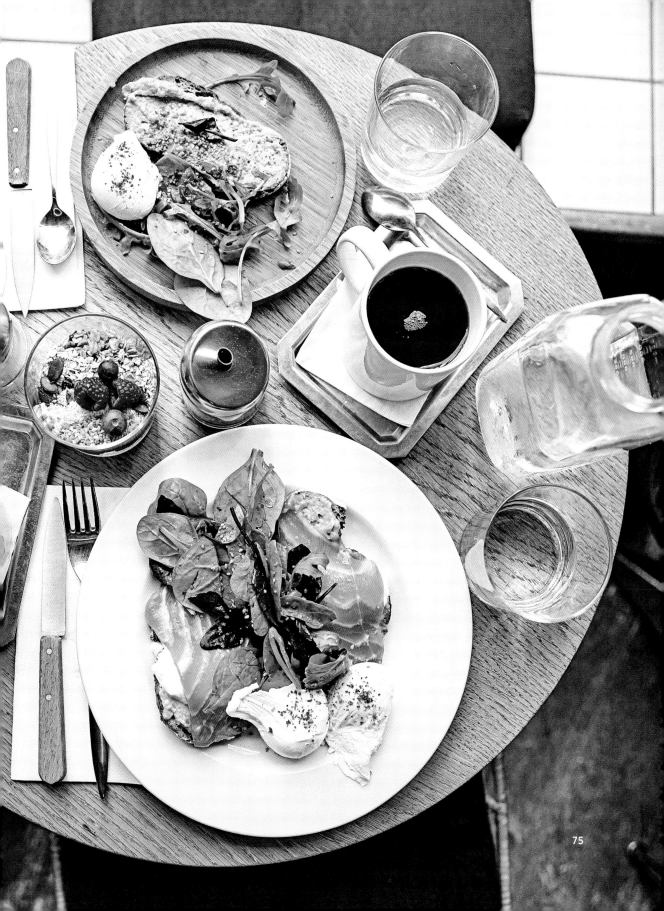

what, when and how you can eat, things are much easier. When you're out and about, you might not be finding anything. Stress comes into play. Many people just abandon it and go back to their usual eating habits." Luckily, with the right prep, that doesn't have to be you.

Before You Head Out of Town

Nuts, hard-boiled eggs and prepacked snacks, like nut butters and bars, are your friends. If you're not going far or are traveling for a short period, don't discount the possibility of packing and making your own food. This is a particularly good option if you're headed somewhere that has a fridge and stove. Though you'll spend additional time in preparation, knowing you have a trove of the right foods ready to go offers ease of mind while traveling. "Those little egg muffins that you can bake are great for this," says Leandro Pucci, M.S., C.N.S., a certified nutrition specialist and integrative health practitioner in West Hollywood, California. "I like to think about it the way my mother would: 'We're going on a field trip; let's pack for the trip.' "

Any holiday travel plan should include making sure you have a healthy collection of snacks. "Whole Foods Market is often my first stop when I'm out of town," says Mavridis. "I grab foods that are calorie-dense and high in protein so I know there's always something that I can eat."

Restaurant Options

Navigating restaurant menus doesn't have to be a nightmare. "Contrary to what many people think, you can eat keto at virtually any restaurant, although some restaurant meals may require some modifications, like replacing a potato with a side salad,"

EXPERTS SAY YOU CAN EAT CARBS AND STILL BE KETO, IF YOU DO SO CONSCIENTIOUSLY.

says Austin, Texas–based Chris Irvin, M.S., education manager at Perfect Keto and co-author of *Keto Answers*.

Irvin recommends keeping your meal simple by sticking to a meat option and a non-starchy vegetable side. Think: steak with a double side of vegetables at an Italian restaurant, or carnitas and a side of guacamole at a Mexican restaurant. To avoid oils like canola, corn or peanut, which aren't keto-compliant, Irvin suggests asking to have your meat or veggies cooked in butter. Or hold the oil altogether and bring your own. "Carry a little bottle of MCT or olive oil," Pucci suggests. "You can put that on a salad and it will help you feel full faster."

Naturally, temptation can be at its peak when you're surrounded by foods you formerly craved. Scope out the restaurant's menu ahead of time and make a game plan so you'll minimize the choices you face when dining out. "If you're eating with other keto dieters, you can also ask the server to hold the bread or chips," Irvin suggests. Be confident about your lifestyle choice, he says, and don't be afraid to make requests.

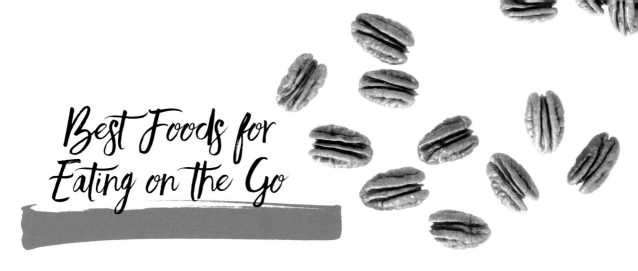

Best Foods for Eating on the Go

✳ Nuts and Nut Butters Look for macadamias, pecans and pili nuts—these nuts have the highest amount of fat and the lowest amount of carbs.

✳ Beef Jerky You can find beef jerky in practically any convenience store. Make sure to select an option that's 100 percent sugar-free. Grass-fed is best when possible.

✳ Chicharróns (aka pork rinds) If you're craving that crunch, chicharróns are your go-to. You'll find them in the chip aisle, but they're packed with protein and 100 percent carb-free.

✳ Charcuterie Go ahead and say "pass the prosciutto" along with the salami, pepperoni and any other cured meat. As long as it's free from sugar, charcuterie is a great option. If you're somewhere a little less fancy, smoked turkey or ham slices work just as well.

✳ Cheese On keto, cheese is permissible in moderate amounts. For maximum flavor, go for aged cheeses but avoid anything orange, as it likely contains artificial colors.

✳ Canned Fish Aside from being delicious, canned fish is high in healthy omega-3 fatty acids, which support brain health.

✳ Olives You can now find olives in ready-to-go single-serve pouches. Because they're primarily made up of healthy monounsaturated fats, olives are an awesome keto snack.

To Carb Cycle or Not to Carb Cycle?

Is there a way to eat carbohydrates now and then and still be on a ketogenic diet? Yes, say the experts.

Carb cycling is a way to strategically cycle a few more carbohydrates in and out of your diet than you would usually eat while adhering to keto. "When you carb cycle, you keep your carb intake low for a set period and then strategically increase carbs to meet a specific health goal," Irvin says. Because increasing carbohydrates floods the body with glucose, which it readily burns as fuel, traditionally that health goal is performance-related: Athletes on a low-carbohydrate diet might carb cycle before high-intensity training days, athletic events or to maintain a certain percentage of body fat. For more details on how to design a holiday-friendly carb-cycling plan, see page 78.

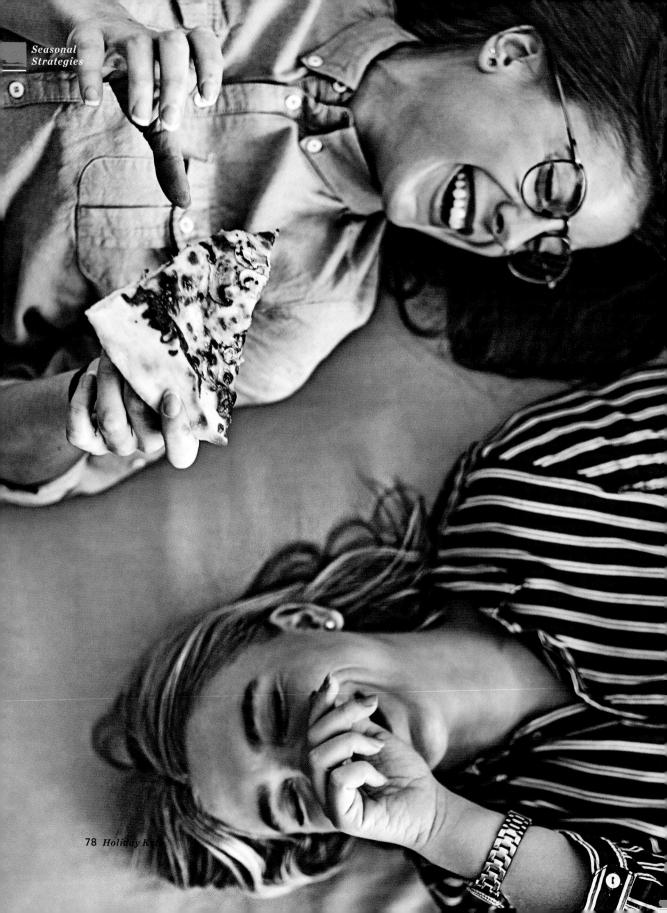

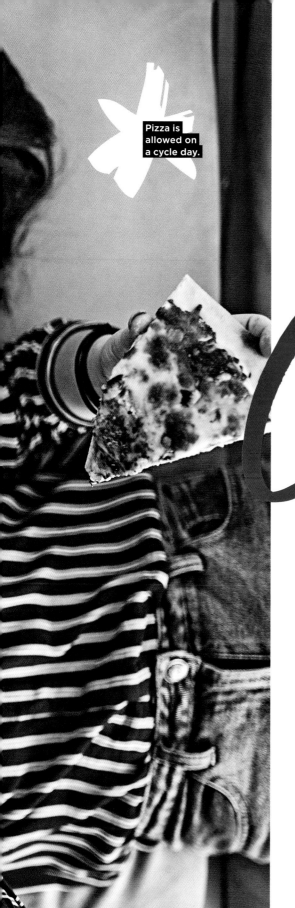

Pizza is allowed on a cycle day.

THE
Cycle
PLAN

Fed up with temptation?
One way to power your way through the holidays is to follow a keto cycling plan, which gives you an occasional breather.

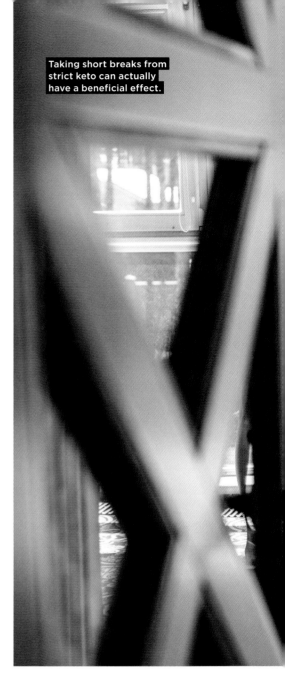

Taking short breaks from strict keto can actually have a beneficial effect.

Keto has a reputation for strictness; after all, keeping carbs at 20 to 50 grams a day knocks a lot of foods off the menu. A plan that restrictive can be even more challenging in a period when you're constantly faced with pies, stuffing and sweets. That's why some experts advise being counterintuitive and taking a day off. It's not actually a "cheat"— it's a technique, says Julie Upton, R.D., co-founder of the nutrition communications firm Appetite for Health. It's called carb cycling, and it involves planning ahead— and indulging in a healthy, not guilty, way.

"What you do is cycle in and out of ketosis, enjoying a more balanced diet on your 'days off,'" Upton explains. It's up to you how you organize your cycling, she adds. Some people do five days of strict keto followed by two non-keto days; others do a six days to one day ratio. "You could also do three weeks on and then a few days off," says Upton. "Many people find they can't stay on keto every single day for too long without taking a break. If you know that break is coming in a few days, or next week, it can help you stick to keto in the short term."

How to Do It

Classic keto breaks down to 75 percent fat, 15 to 20 percent protein, and 5 to 10 percent carbs. On a "cycle" day, you change those macro proportions to about 25 percent fat, 25 percent protein and 50 percent carbs. During the holidays, you could "let up" a bit on a day when you have a cocktail party—or even for Thanksgiving.

One key to making carb cycling work, though, is to not fall into a binge. A cycle day doesn't mean two pieces of pie and loads of stuffing. Instead, says Upton, "eat wholesome carb-rich foods." Rather than a marshmallow-topped sweet potato casserole, treat yourself to a baked sweet potato with butter. After being on keto, you'll be amazed at how sugary that will taste. Other good choices: fruits, whole grains (say, a warm bowl of oatmeal), and starchy veggies like corn or beets.

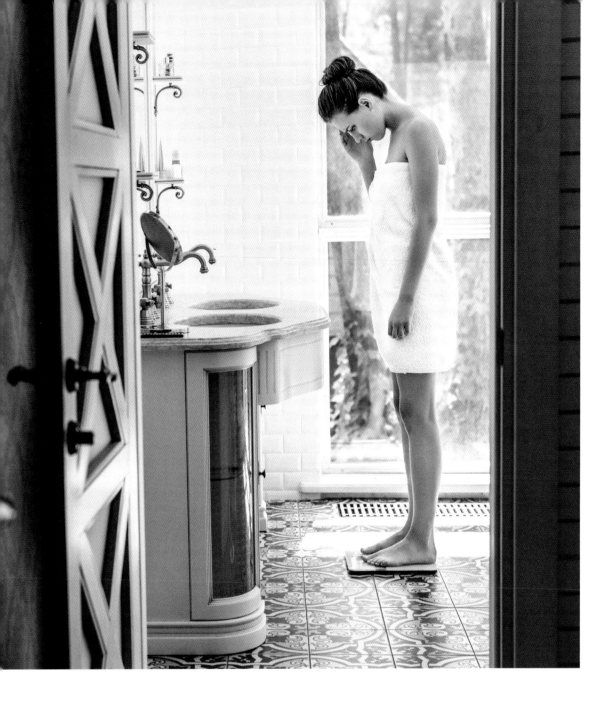

Insider Tips

To avoid too many fluctuations on the scale, some people opt to pump up their exercise program on cycle days, says Upton. And a few extra carbs can give you an energy bump before a workout. But remember, those fluctuations likely will happen, so don't panic. Carbs hold water in the cells, and that alone can add a few pounds. But once you're back to keto and in ketosis again, your weight will stabilize. The wisest course is to step away from the scale for a few days after your cycle day—and remind yourself that cycling may have helped you stick to keto long-term.

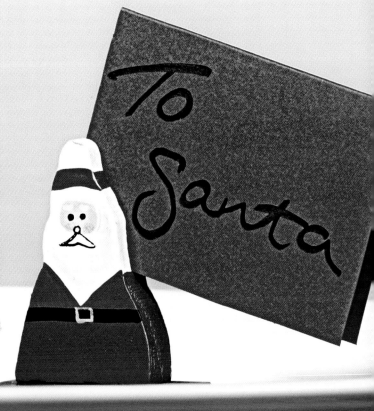

Just a Taste! "Cheating" can be a learning experience.

To Santa

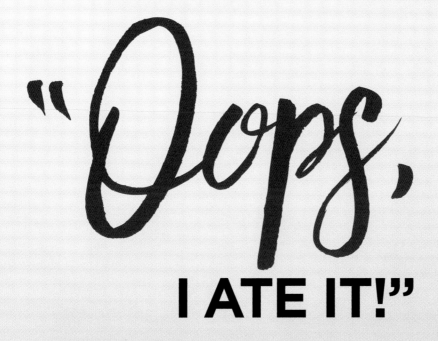

"Oops,
I ATE IT!"

News flash: Nobody's perfect. Here's how to bounce back when you've broken your own rules.

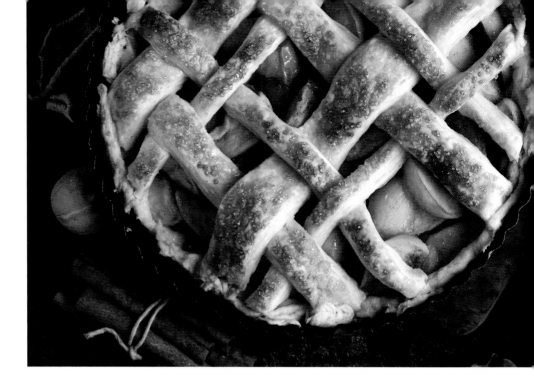

You caved in to the pie. You sneaked extra stuffing. First of all, there's enough guilt around food and eating already, so try not to beat yourself up. "You don't have to be perfect on the diet to experience real change and improvements in your health," says Josh Axe, D.N.M., founder of Ancient Nutrition and *draxe.com,* and author of *Keto Diet*. "Keto has powerful effects on your metabolism, so a slipup here and there doesn't mean you won't make any progress and should call it quits."

But what should you do? What's the script for getting back on track? Here's a (mostly) painless guide to picking up where you left off.

Don't Punish Yourself

The worst thing you can do is "discipline" yourself by hardly eating anything, says Katherine Brooking, M.S., R.D., co-founder of *appforhealth.com.* That's sure to prompt more angst, not to mention hunger—which could well boomerang into overeating later, or even another trip past the dessert table. Go right back to your usual routine at the next meal, and forget about trying to "make up for" your misstep by starving yourself.

Identify Triggers

"Ask yourself, 'Was it the holiday food? Stress? Boredom? That the diet feels too restrictive?'" suggests Brooking. "Then you can take action to deal with the underlying issues." For instance, the holiday period is notoriously stressful and overscheduled. Resolve to give yourself some solid "me time," and try to work in some exercise or meditation, both effective stress-busters.

Get Cooking

If you decide the problem is the greater temptations of holiday foods, or that you have limited what you eat too strictly, rethink your approach to keto. Some people fall into a habit of eating simply chicken and salad, or fish and vegetables; suddenly, what everyone else is having looks so much better. Look up some new keto-friendly

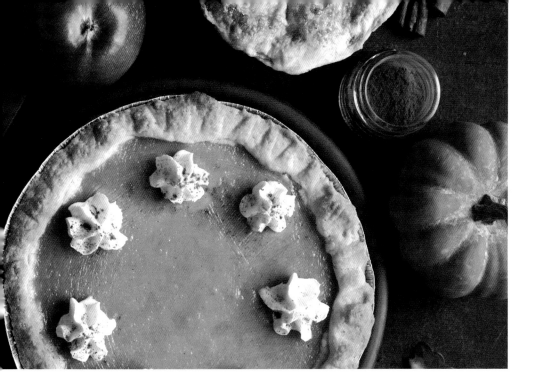

recipes and broaden your repertoire. There are many ways to make keto versions of what you're craving—breads, pies, cookies—so you can satisfy that sweet tooth without going on a carb binge.

Prep for Next Time

Map out ways you'll deal with future temptations, says Andreas Eenfeldt, M.D., founder of *dietdoctor.com*. One good technique is the simple delay tactic. "If you're tempted to eat dessert at a dinner party, tell yourself, 'I'll wait and have some dark chocolate when I get home instead.' Later, at home, that moment has passed and your food environment has changed—you're not watching friends inhale dessert." (And, of course, if you still want it, a square of dark chocolate is permissible on keto!) Similarly, you see a croissant or pastry on the breakfast buffet and want to dive in; tell yourself you can eat it, but not until you've had the rest of your breakfast. After eggs and bacon, the urge probably will have passed.

Especially during the holidays, when temptations abound, make sure you carry low-carb snacks like walnuts, macadamia nuts or Babybel cheeses with you. In the middle of a hectic holiday shopping trip, you're more likely to give in to a food-court nosh of pizza or a hot dog, but the right snack can derail the cravings.

Consider a Cheat

There are good and bad reasons to plan a quick "cheat," says Eenfeldt. Bad reasons include impulse (you won't really enjoy those cold French fries your kid didn't finish, or that dry slice of office birthday cake) and being polite or wanting to fit in—people don't really care as much as you think! Less-bad reasons include a thoughtful decision to take advantage of a rare opportunity. "Your favorite dessert, a special pumpkin pie made just once a year by a dear family friend...this could be a time to make an exception to your no-dessert rule," Eenfeldt says. Enjoy every bite, and then get back on the keto wagon.

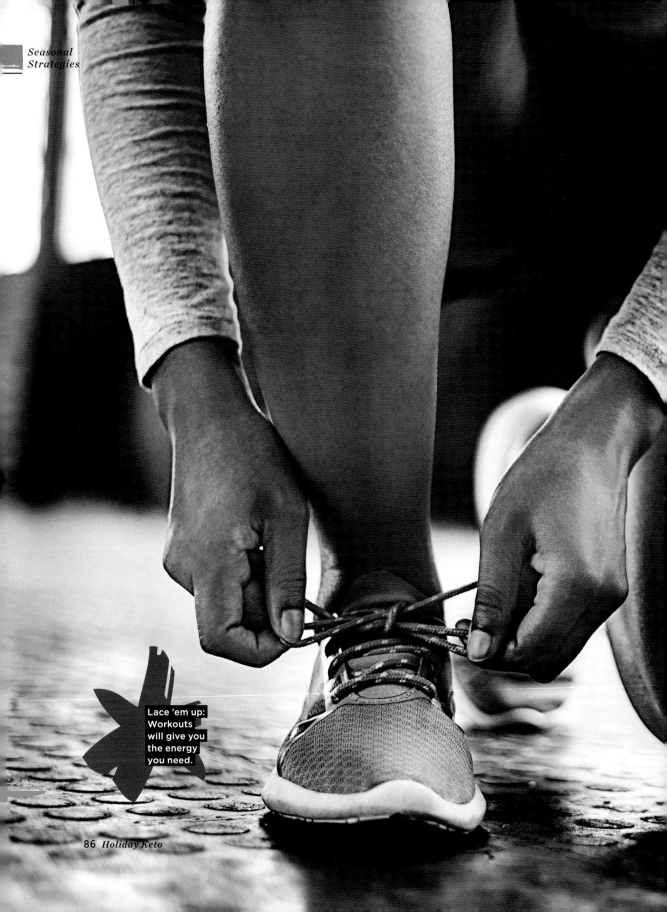

Lace 'em up:
Workouts
will give you
the energy
you need.

THE
Stay-Fit
HOLIDAY
PLAN

Yes, you're busy...and frazzled...and tense. And these are all reasons to give yourself the gift of sticking with— or starting—an exercise program to keep you on the keto track!

The No. 1 excuse for skipping exercise—"I don't have the time!"—feels even more respectable in November and December. The days are getting shorter, you've put away swimsuits and pulled out big sweaters, and you're mapping out parties, festive dinners and gift-buying. But there's another truth about exercise: It's been documented to reduce stress and improve both confidence and mood—all benefits that come in extra handy in these crowded days.

OK, but how do you get around to it? And where do you find the motivation? "We all lie to ourselves and say we don't have the time," says Ramsey Bergeron, a trainer, keto triathlete and owner of Bergeron Personal Training in Scottsdale, Arizona. "But it's not about having the time, it's about making the time—even just 30 minutes." Check out these insider insights for squeezing in exercise.

Practice Little Tricks

Let's say you're doing a lot of shopping. Park farther away and walk to the stores, says Bergeron. "You might actually get to the store more quickly by not circling around looking for a close spot," he adds. At home, work in little moves during the day. When you're standing in the kitchen stirring things on the stove, "practice squeezing your glutes together," says Bergeron. "You'll be surprised how effective it is, especially if you tend to sit too much during the day." You can also take little "squat breaks" to work thighs and glutes while you're waiting for pots to boil or the timer to ring.

To reduce tension, which often expresses itself as back or neck pain, take a few minutes to do some stretches to release your muscles. If you've been standing for a long time—in the kitchen or in line to pay at stores—your lower back can tighten up. Do a few sitting or standing hamstring stretches, along with simple yoga poses like downward-facing dog and cobra. Another quickie: While watching TV, use the ad breaks to do a plank (see how long you can hold it) or a set of push-ups.

Do Compound Moves

This is a great way to compress your workouts into less time, says Bergeron. Rather than working one group of muscles at a time—say, your quads or delts—double up by doing moves that work several muscle groups. "Compound movements use at least two joints," explains Bergeron. "For instance, a bench press, which moves at the shoulder and the elbow, is much more effective than just doing curls."

Some examples: Do lunges with bicep curls worked in, and squats or step-ups with overhead presses. Also, some moves are compound simply because they engage so many parts of the body. Consider deadlifts, in which you lift a weight from the floor to a standing position by hinging forward at the waist; this works the glutes, hamstrings, core and upper-, mid- and lower-back muscles. That's a lot of targets in one move. One of the simplest compound exercises of all is the push-up, which uses the arms, shoulders, core, serratus (muscles at the sides of your ribs) and chest, along with the legs, glutes and lats—talk about multitasking!

Shorten Your Aerobic Workouts

This may be music to most people's ears—but it's also proven to be just as effective as longer, endurance-style workouts. More evidence, including a meta-analysis this year in *The British Journal of Sports Medicine*, points to the benefits of high-intensity interval training (HIIT). These

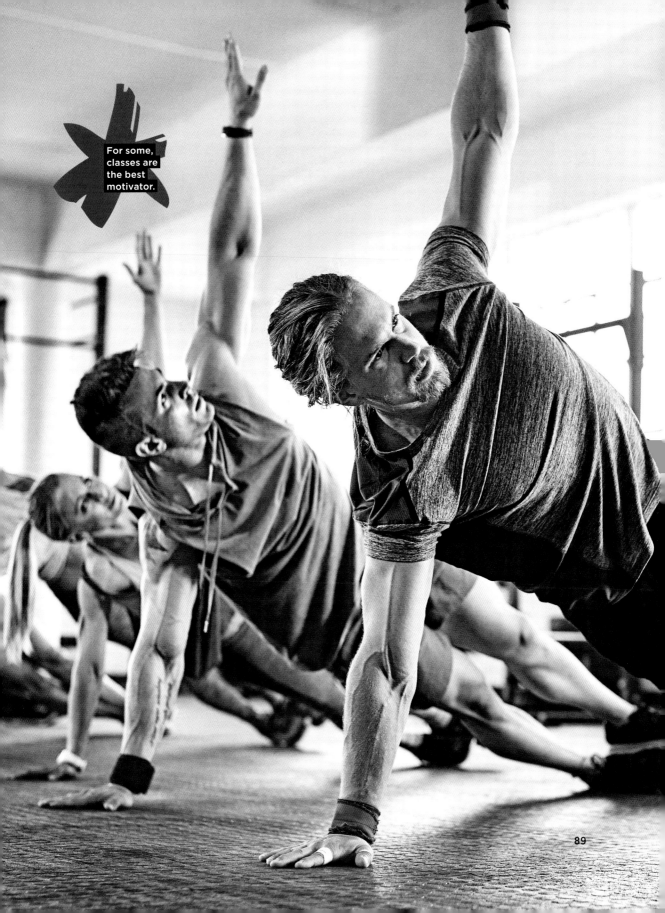

For some, classes are the best motivator.

89

workouts can last only 15, 20 or at most 30 minutes, and they combine very short periods of all-out effort, like a sprint, with longer recovery periods at a moderate effort. The recent study found that not only is HIIT just as good for your health as a 40-minute, moderately paced run, but that interval training can even burn more fat than a long walk or jog.

To get the best of both worlds during a time when you're super busy, try doing a 15-minute run or bike ride with high-intensity intervals, along with 15 minutes of compound weight-lifting moves. Another way to speed up benefits, says Bergeron: Instead of doing a "legs day" or an "upper-body day," combine both in an alternating pattern. So at the gym you might do one set of lat pull-downs to work the back, then switch to a leg-press machine and do one set that targets thighs and glutes. Then return to the first move and repeat. "This allows one part of your body to rest while another part is working, which can shorten your time in the gym," Bergeron says.

Get an Early Start

Face it: If you plan to squeeze in a workout "sometime today," it probably won't happen. "If you want to stick to a workout routine, you have to schedule it," says Bergeron. And increasing evidence shows that morning workouts may be not only the most likely to occur, but perhaps be more effective. A 2019 study published in *The International Journal of Obesity* followed 100 people over 10 months as they committed to working out five days a week. They all did the same exercises, burning 600 calories at each workout, and almost all of them lost weight. But the people who exercised before noon

Stress Relief
Studies show that any exercise can boost your mood.

lost more weight than those who did the same workouts later in the day, after 3 p.m.

That's quite an incentive to get up a tiny bit earlier. And one other element has been shown to boost your benefits: skipping breakfast. A 2019 study in *The Journal of Nutrition* showed that people who worked out first thing on an empty stomach and didn't eat until lunch took in fewer calories during the day. It may be that when you exercise before eating, your body has to rely on stored energy—and if you're ketogenic, that means stored fats and ketones. That makes you hungrier in the short term, and the people in the study ate a larger lunch than those who had breakfasted before working out. But by the end of the day, they took in 400 fewer calories than the breakfast eaters, so their spike in hunger for lunch was urgent but short-lived.

Work Out at Home

Sometimes the thought of getting to the gym—or to the track on a cold morning—dampens the workout urge. So...don't leave the house. There is a plethora of exercise routines available on DVD or that can be downloaded or streamed. You save the time of going to the gym, and you can finish your workout in a half-hour total. Some favorites: **BBG by Kayla Itsines:** The Bikini Body Guide series incorporates low-intensity cardio, high-intensity interval training and strength-training circuit workouts that challenge your muscles. (*kaylaitsines.com*) **PIIT 28:** This is a 28-day Pilates-based interval training program that combines core-strengthening exercises with high-intensity interval training routines to create PIIT, which stands for Pilates Intense Interval Training. (*piit28.com*)

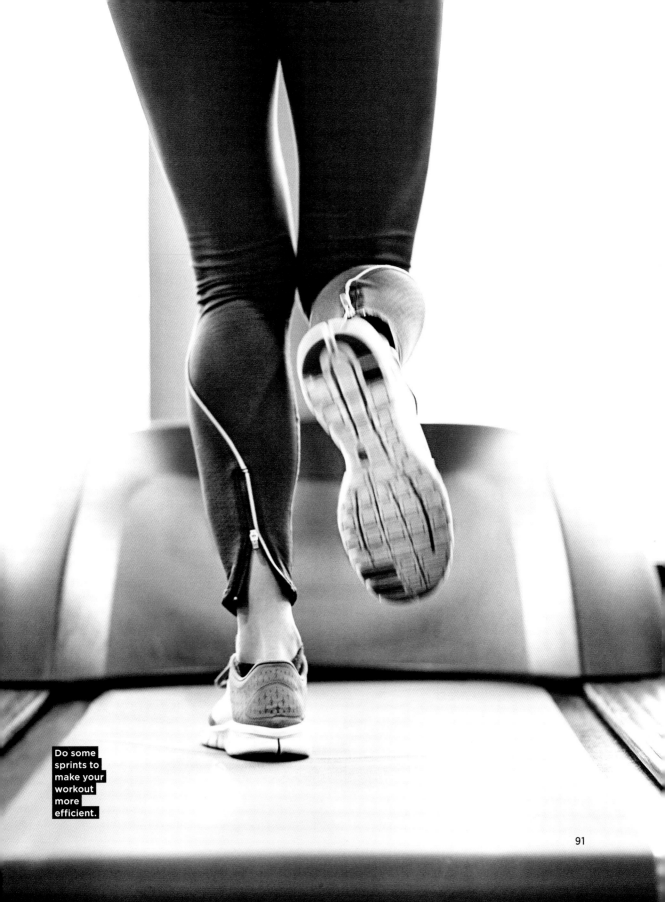

Do some sprints to make your workout more efficient.

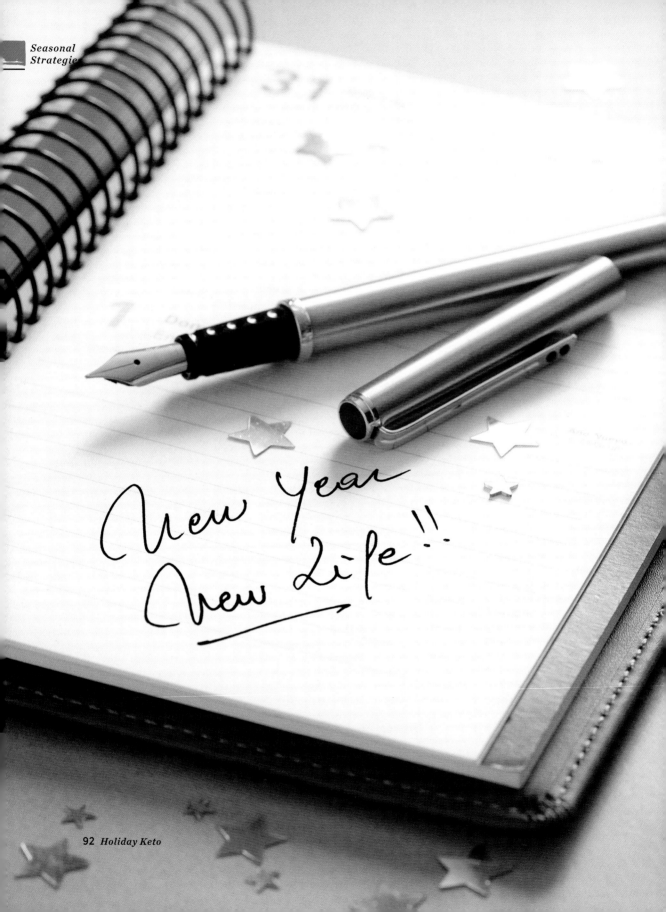

READY
SET
Goals!

Discover the tools and tactics
you need to make your experience
with keto a success.

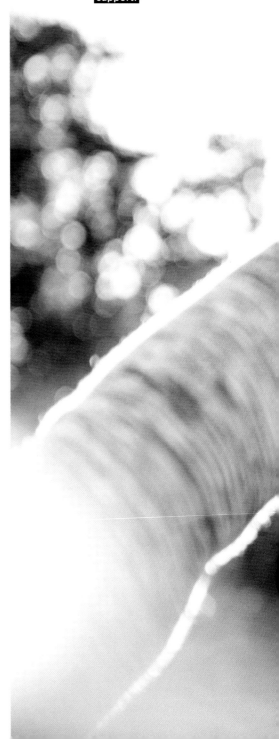

You don't have to go it alone: Join a group for some extra support.

The words "I'm on a diet" are rarely accompanied by a smile, and for good reason. Not only has the word "diet" become associated with negatives like restriction and deprivation, but many experts have concluded that a majority of dieters will gain back all the weight they've lost within three to five years. In fact, the authors of a 2007 study at UCLA concluded that most dieters "would have been better off not going on a diet at all."

Pretty depressing, right? But what if you could reframe going on the keto diet? Why not think of it as a long-term lifestyle change rather than a short-term, quick-fix solution? According to Birmingham, Alabama–based personal trainer Lauren Floyd, that could be the key to success. She also says we need to chill out. "That may seem counterintuitive, since the majority of us are looking for ways to 'get our butt in gear' and 'stop being couch potatoes,'" she says. "But in a lot of ways our culture's overly rigid, black-and-white approach to 'health' and 'actualization' is what's causing many of the issues we see around body-image dissatisfaction, cyclical weight gain/loss, lack of motivation and energy, general feelings of exhaustion, and stress or anxiety over not being enough and burnout."

Making the decision to adopt a new lifestyle isn't easy, but we've got some tips and tricks that will help you stay the course and achieve your weight-loss and better-health goals, even during the holidays.

Reevaluate Your Relationship with Food

"Food doesn't have a moral value, so don't separate foods into 'good' or 'bad,'" says Floyd. "Think of food as a fuel for your body that comes in different grades of calories

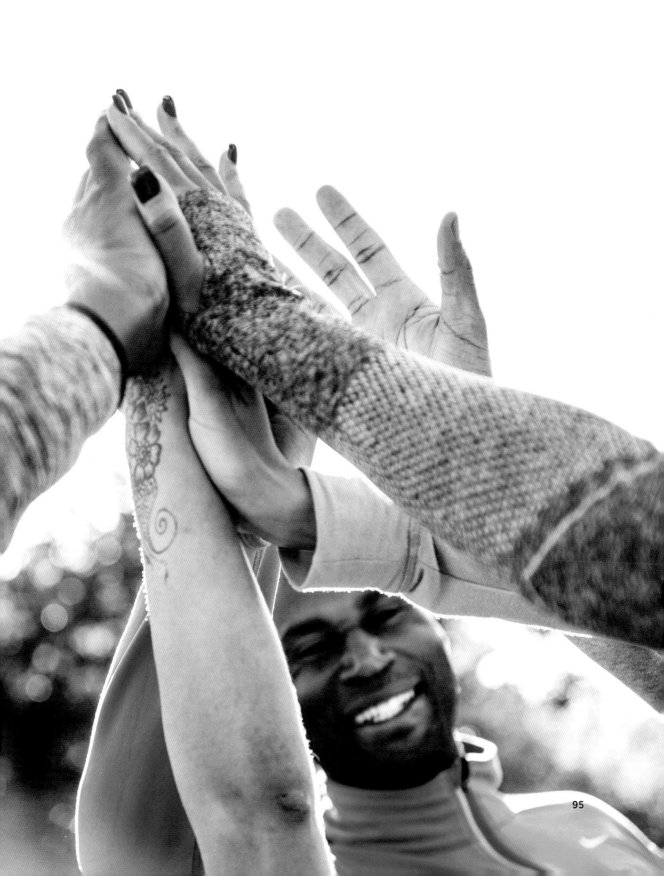

and nutrients—basic, plus and superior. All foods give you energy, but not all of them will give it to you in the most effective way." Do your homework—or even consider working with a nutritionist—to come up with a long list of meal and snack options, so you can always have your necessary fats, carbs and proteins at the ready. You're less likely to "cheat" if you have meals prepped and ready to go.

Choose an Exercise That You Enjoy

A healthy lifestyle includes exercise. The Mayo Clinic recommends that adults get at least 150 minutes of moderate or 75 minutes of vigorous exercise per week in addition to strength-training twice a week. So it's time to stop thinking of exercise as a punishment or an activity you have to endure. But if you really hate running, don't make running your exercise of choice because you're going to spend more time looking for excuses than actually running. Test the waters: Try a dance class with holiday music, take a walk and check out the neighborhood holiday decorations, try yoga. Then make sure you keep up the good work! "Our bodies are meant to move, and when we do, we're rewarded with serotonin and endorphins," Floyd adds.

Use Mantras

Words have power. When you're having a moment of weakness and want to trade keto for cake or a cookie, pep yourself up with simple phrases like, "One day at a time," "I am enough," or "Do the next best thing." You can also give yourself a time-out when you get overwhelmed. Take a five-minute break to concentrate on your breathing or take a few moments to drink an extra glass of water.

WORDS HAVE POWER. THE WAY WE SPEAK TO OURSELVES DICTATES OUR ACTIONS AND OUTCOMES.

Take Baby Steps Toward Your Goals

Patience is a virtue. It's best that you accept that you can't accomplish everything in one day. Start small. Begin each day by making one choice that supports your overall goal. "After a couple of days of making one choice to get what you want, progress to making two choices that support your goal, and so on. And when you 'mess up' or 'fall off the wagon' for a day, don't freak out! Have some self-compassion and pick up where you left off," says Floyd.

Write Down Your Accomplishments

Instead of concentrating on all the "should haves" and "could haves" each night, give yourself a pat on the back and write down all the "right" things—no matter how small they may seem—you chose to do that supported your bigger goal. You might be surprised at how effectively this ritual can help keep you on track, and the journal entries will likely be inspirational later on in your journey.

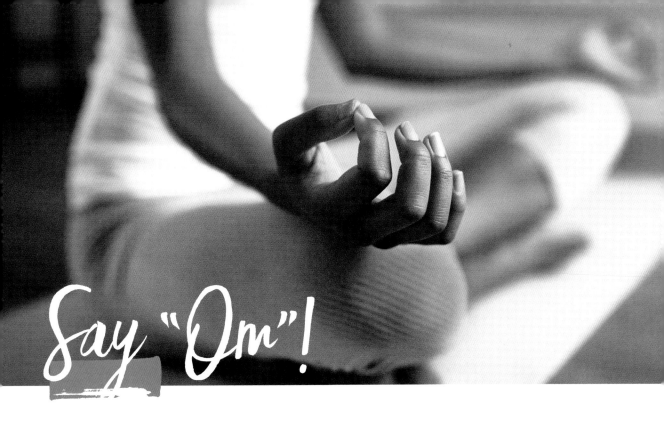

Say "Om"!

You already possess a powerful weapon that will help you accomplish your keto goals: your mind. On those days when you think you're too stressed, too busy or too mad to stick with it, look to "mindfulness"—observing your thoughts and feelings without judging them. A meditative state can help reduce stress, boost memory, sharpen focus and, yes, help you achieve your goals—and it doesn't require hours on end. Here, four simple ways to get yourself in the right frame of mind no matter what the season may bring.

DEEP BREATHS
"Beginning each morning with a breathing exercise can really set the tone for the day," says yoga and mindfulness teacher Georgette Dunn of Ready.Set.Flow in Dallas. She suggests breathing in and out slowly. One breath cycle should last for approximately six seconds. "Breathe in through your nose and out through your mouth, letting your breath flow effortlessly in and out of your body," Dunn adds.

SLOW DOWN
Eat your meal slowly and really connect to the ways it is benefiting your body, Dunn suggests. This intention can help steer you toward good food choices. The practice of mindful eating—being fully aware—comes from Buddhism, and can help you slow down. "Focus intentionally on your food, noticing all sensation and taking in the flavors, textures, smells and colors," says Meredith Milton, a Seattle-based nutritionist and mindful eating coach.

YAWN
Mindfulness is the opposite of day-dreaming or dozing off, so it might seem a bit surprising that there's an exercise that calls for you to make yourself yawn—and not from chowing down on all that Thanksgiving turkey! Even an artificial yawn can bring you into the here and now—and optimize metabolism. Take a slow, deep breath followed by a yawn, while paying attention to the sensations. Follow it up with a very slow stretching session for at least 30 seconds.

ONE THING AT A TIME
Lay off the multi-tasking. When you're doing keto food prep, say, focus on that food prep. When you're going for a walk, focus on your steps not your incoming texts. Says Dunn: "Take on each task with full awareness, one by one. When you're mindful of what you're doing, you're less prone to rushing, making mistakes or forgetting details. You'll probably find you can be more efficient and finish the task without feeling frustrated or tense."

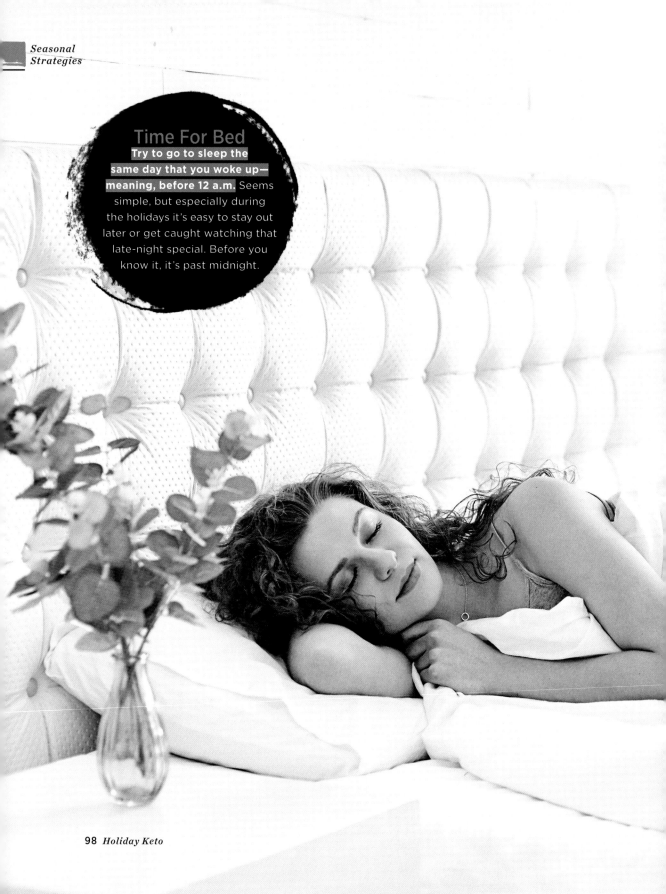

Time For Bed

Try to go to sleep the same day that you woke up—meaning, before 12 a.m. Seems simple, but especially during the holidays it's easy to stay out later or get caught watching that late-night special. Before you know it, it's past midnight.

What's Sleep

GOT TO DO WITH IT?

There's more to shut-eye than feeling refreshed.
Catching 40 winks (or more!) supports a healthy lifestyle,
especially during festive times.

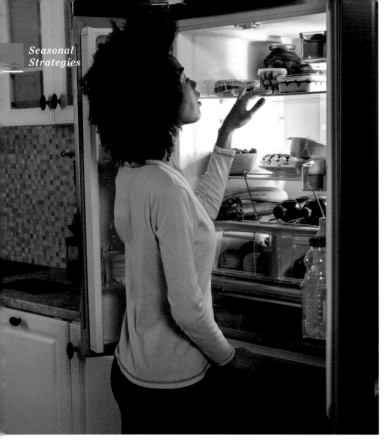

Healthy Eating When
You're Tired

It's no coincidence: When we're sleep-deprived, levels of the appetite-stimulating hormone ghrelin increase, while levels of leptin—the hormone that suppresses appetite—fall. This makes us feel more hungry. But that's not the only thing that happens. Sleep deprivation also raises the blood level of compounds in the body that make eating junk food (and all that holiday candy) all the more enjoyable. The National Sleep Foundation reports that people who don't get enough sleep eat twice as much fat—and more than 300 extra calories—the next day, compared with those who sleep for eight hours.

You might think holidays like Thanksgiving, Christmas and New Year's are times when people can catch up on sleep. But it's not so. Parents, especially, drink more and sleep less. And studies show that sleep deprivation is associated with obesity and weight gain, cognitive decline, and hormone and blood sugar imbalances. It can even put us on a path to other chronic illnesses. The problem is, many of us know this but still don't get enough sleep! The National Institutes of Health recommends that adults older than 18 get seven to nine hours of sleep each night, which is about 49 to 63 hours of sleep per week. The reality? Studies show that 40 percent of adults are falling short of that minimum of 49. And during the holidays, that percentage can rise to more than 50 percent. If this is you, now is a good time to start tracking your sleep to see how much you're really getting. And when the holidays arrive with all their tasty temptations, it's even more important for your health to make sure you're getting a sufficient amount of rest.

How to Get the Zzz's You Need

Too stressed about gift-buying and all you have to do during the season to sleep well? Follow these tips to help you relax and get a night of restful slumber.

1 Exercise Daily Done early in the day, it can improve your sleep quality, according to the National Sleep Foundation. Working out not only helps to ward off stress but it also increases the body's temperature by a few degrees. Later in the day, as your body's temperature drops back down to its normal range, this change can bring on drowsiness, which will help you nod off.

2 Cut off Caffeine Aim to have your last caffeinated beverage of the day by 3 p.m. if you're having difficulty sleeping. Drinking alcohol at night can also have a negative effect on your rest, so skip the spiked eggnog. Eating a clean diet (like keto) is thought to help improve sleep.

3 Turn off the Technology This includes your computer, phone, the TV—anything with a screen, especially as bedtime nears. The blue and green light emitted by these devices interferes with the natural effects of the sleep-promoting hormone melatonin.

4 Take a Warm Shower or Bath It will help you to relax before hopping into bed. Sipping chamomile tea can also help you unwind.

5 Try Aromatherapy Some scents have been shown to promote relaxation. Spray your pillow with a scented mist like lavender or jasmine, or place calming essential oils in a diffuser or dab them across your forehead.

6 Get Comfy Make sure you have a pillow that's the right firmness for your neck and sheets that you absolutely love.

7 Try Meditating Before Sleep Even if it's just for five to 10 minutes, clearing your mind can help calm your nervous system and help you let go of the day's stressors so they don't rumble around in your mind while you're trying to snooze.

8 Keep a Journal by Your Bed If thinking about all the things you need to do the next day is keeping you awake, take a moment to write those things down.

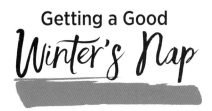

Getting a Good
Winter's Nap

Respondents to a survey conducted by the National Sleep Foundation ranked these elements of their sleep experience as the most important:

✹ Comfortable Mattress
✹ Comfortable Pillows
✹ Comfortable Sheets
✹ Quiet Room
✹ Dark Room
✹ Cool Room Temperature
✹ Fresh Air, Free of Allergens
✹ Clean Bedroom

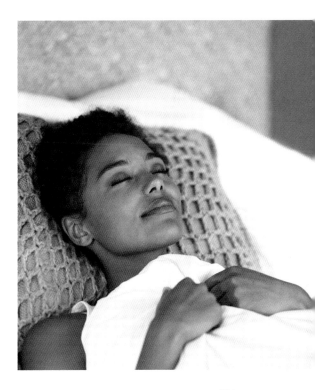

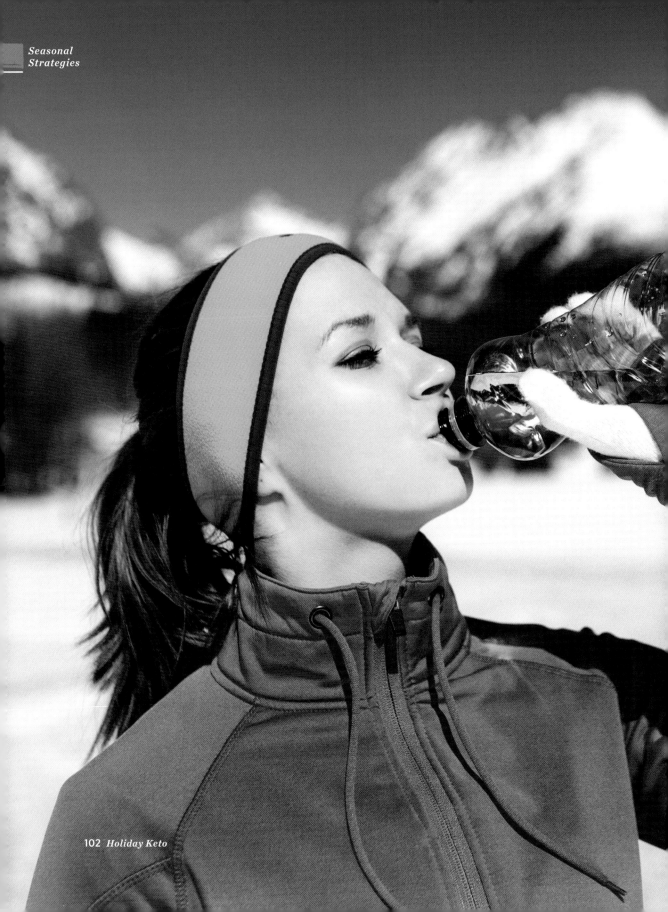

Drink Up!

Water—not holiday cocktails—is a key part of **transitioning to keto with minimal side effects.**

When you first kick off the keto diet, you may notice your pants suddenly feel a whole lot looser. In fact, rapid weight loss is one of the hallmark characteristics of going keto. That's because when you slash carbs from your diet, your body naturally sheds water weight. Carbs are stored in your muscles and liver as glycogen; each gram of glycogen contains about 3 to 4 grams of water. So when your body taps into those glycogen stores for energy, that water weight comes off with it. An estimated 70 percent of weight loss in the first week of a keto diet is due to water weight; over time, as you tap into fat stores, that number will drop significantly.

Losing this much water can not only cause dehydration; it can also throw your body's electrolytes out of balance, which is in part why you might feel symptoms of the keto flu.

"People need sodium, magnesium and potassium when they do a low-carb diet," says Tracey Grant, R.D.N. Adding these electrolytes—or at the very least, salt—can minimize uncomfortable side effects. "If someone is not feeling well, or is light-headed, dizzy or nauseous, I encourage them to look at electrolytes and hydration," she says. Even mild dehydration can zap your energy, memory and attention,

Hydration Equation

Divide your weight by two: That's what you should drink in ounces daily. For instance, if you weigh 160 pounds, then try to take in roughly 80 ounces, or 10 cups, of water. Be sure to include electrolytes in your hydration plan to avoid side effects like the keto flu.

while an electrolyte deficiency can create headaches, weakness and nausea.

Sodium and potassium, in particular, are needed to help maintain adequate fluid levels and blood volume. While you can optimize potassium intake from foods such as avocados and coconuts, if you are having rapid water-weight loss, you may need to augment your intake with a supplement or liquid electrolytes.

Another common side effect of a low-carb diet is constipation, but increasing fluid intake can help keep your digestive system more regular. Plus, staying hydrated helps support the kidneys' role of filtering out unnecessary toxins that can be created through ketosis.

Make proper hydration a daily habit from the start, drinking water or other fluids regularly throughout the day. The best way to remind yourself is to keep a water bottle at your desk or carry one with you. While coffee and tea have a mild diuretic effect, they still count (just avoid the milk and sugar), or eat foods with a higher water content, such as soups and vegetables. And if you're at a party, sip plenty of water along with (or instead of) those festive cocktails.

ELECTROLYTES ARE KEY TO MAKING SURE YOUR NERVES, MUSCLES, HEART AND BRAIN ALL FUNCTION AT THEIR BEST.

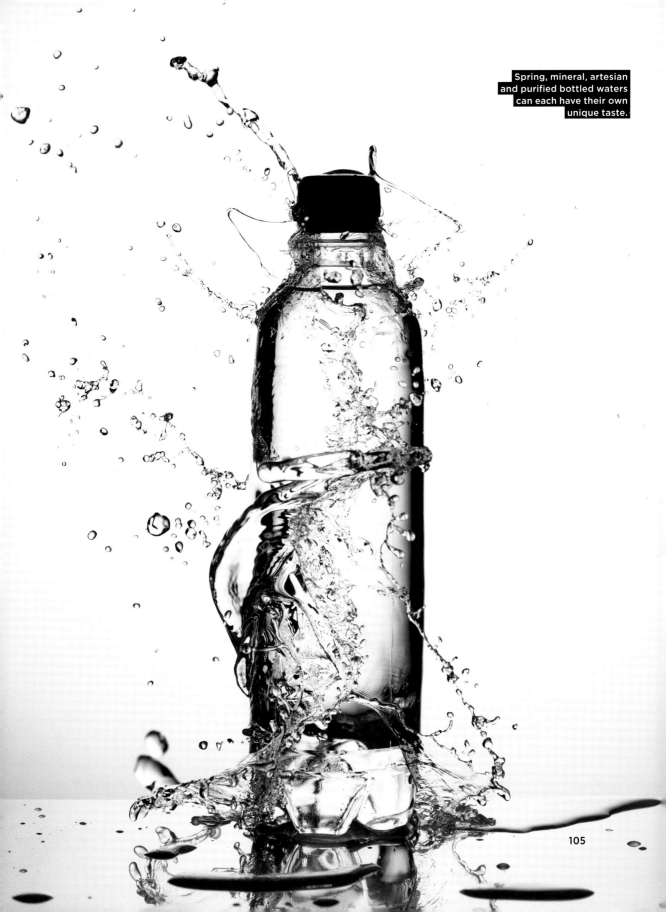

Spring, mineral, artesian and purified bottled waters can each have their own unique taste.

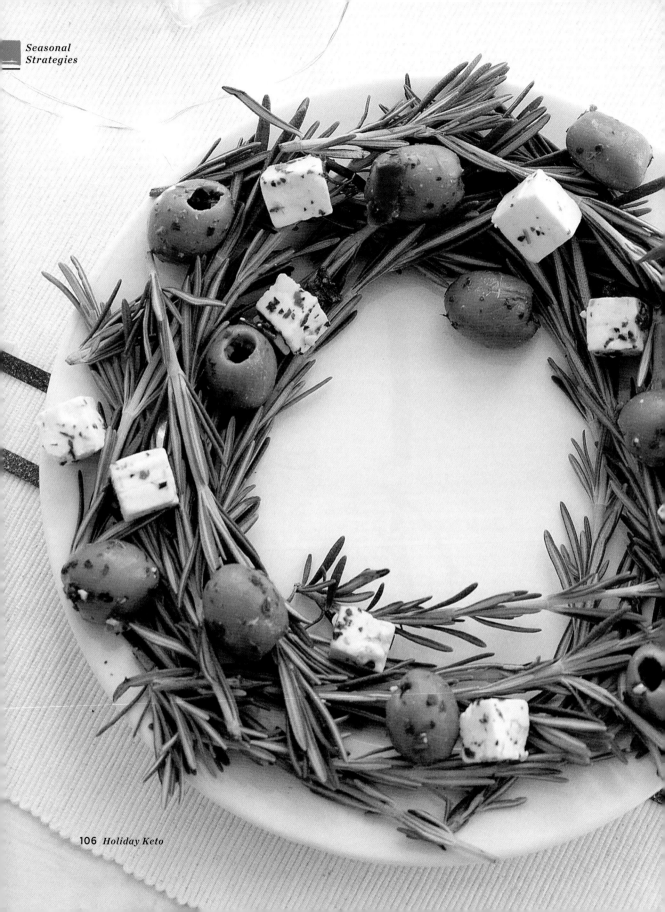

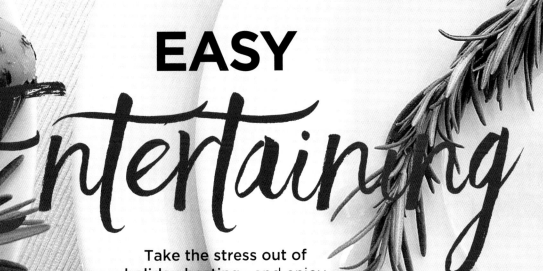

EASY
Entertaining

Take the stress out of holiday hosting—and enjoy your own fiesta—with these essential party tips.

107

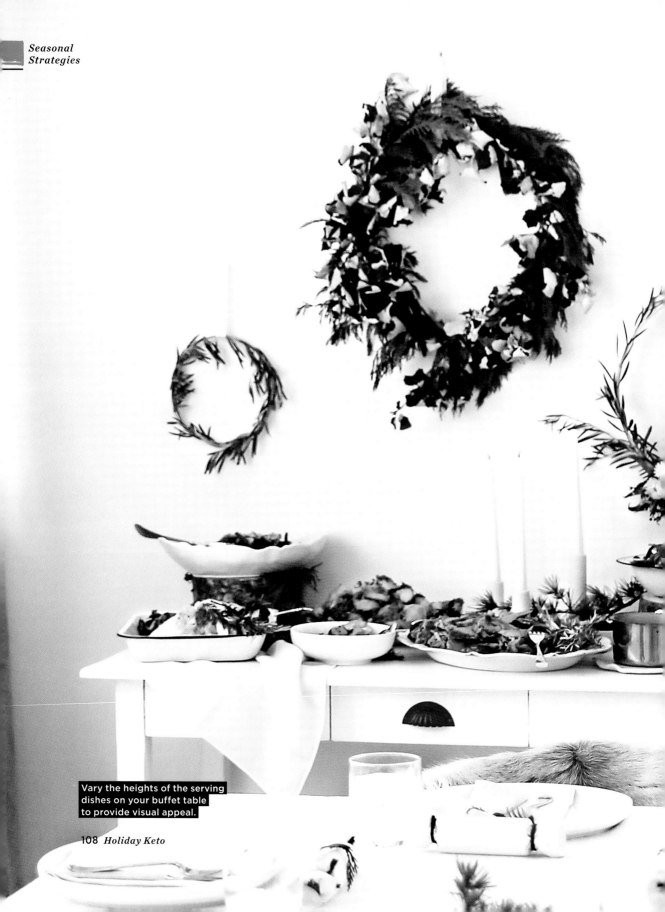

Vary the heights of the serving
dishes on your buffet table
to provide visual appeal.

Buffet Pointers

There's a lot to be said for presenting a holiday dinner as a buffet: It prompts a relaxed, fun atmosphere, and lets people fill their plates according to their tastes. Here's how to ace yours.

1 **Set up the table to move from left to right,** starting with stacks of plates on the left end of the table. Put knives and forks rolled in napkins at the right end. In between, start with the big dish—turkey or other main course—followed by stuffing and casseroles, then veggies and salads.

2 **Put desserts on a separate buffet table,** if you have the space, along with coffee and after-dinner drinks. You can set out many of the desserts ahead of time, but here's a pie tip: Put your pies in a turned-off but still warm oven just before you set out dinner, and they'll be the right temperature when dessert time rolls around.

3 **Label all the dishes.** This will be especially helpful in cluing people in to which buffet items conform to either keto/low-carb or other restrictions, such as gluten-free, vegetarian or vegan. Labels are also helpful as you're setting up, since they make it crystal clear which dishes go where when you (or your helpers) are putting food on the table.

4 **Pre-portion as much of the food as possible.** This both makes it easier for people to serve themselves, and keeps the display looking nicer as people pass through. So, for example, cut casseroles into sections, if possible.

5 **If you're setting out a charcuterie platter, make sure to put out the cheese early**—it's tastiest at room temperature.

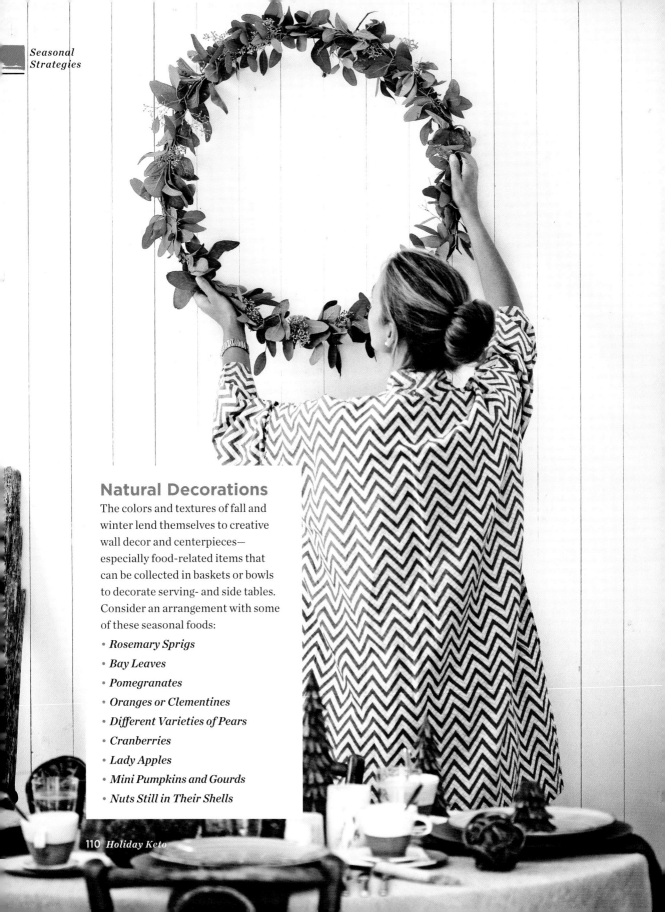

Natural Decorations

The colors and textures of fall and winter lend themselves to creative wall decor and centerpieces—especially food-related items that can be collected in baskets or bowls to decorate serving- and side tables. Consider an arrangement with some of these seasonal foods:

- *Rosemary Sprigs*
- *Bay Leaves*
- *Pomegranates*
- *Oranges or Clementines*
- *Different Varieties of Pears*
- *Cranberries*
- *Lady Apples*
- *Mini Pumpkins and Gourds*
- *Nuts Still in Their Shells*

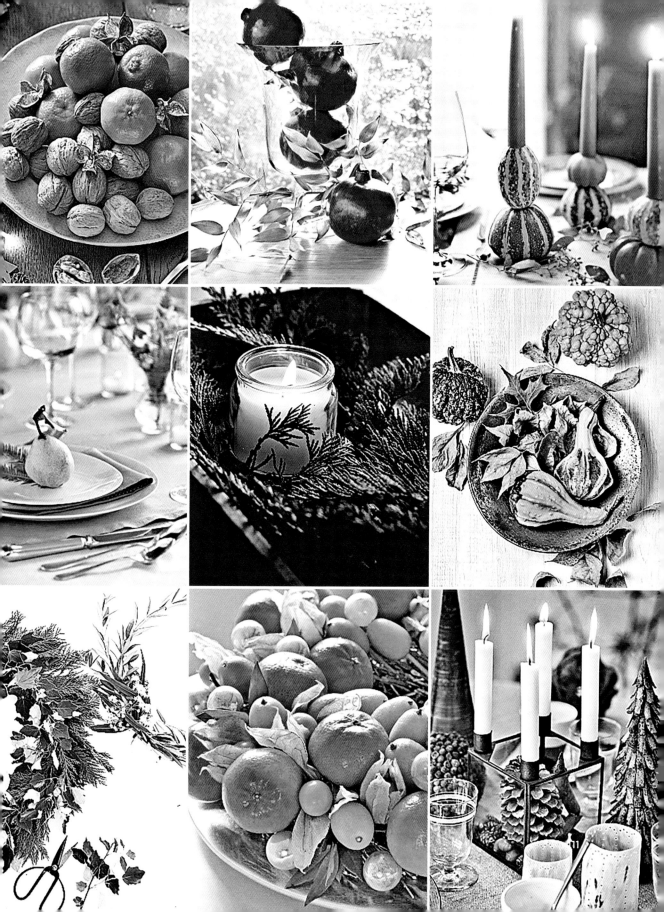

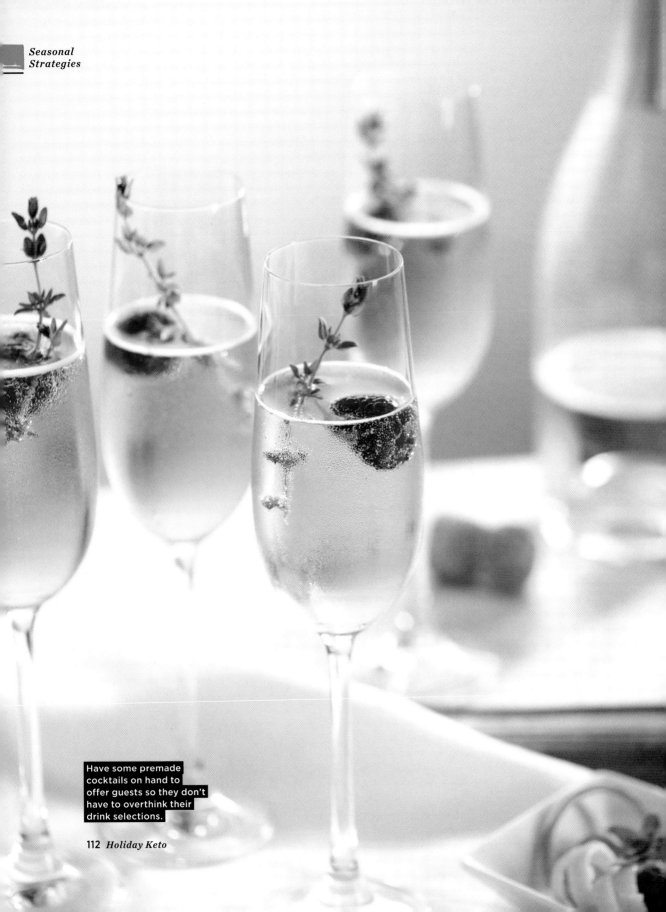

Have some premade
cocktails on hand to
offer guests so they don't
have to overthink their
drink selections.

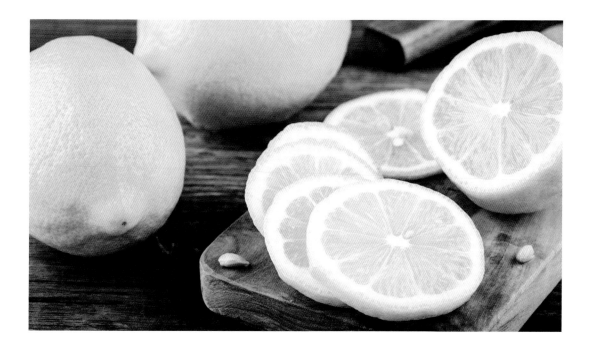

Setting Up a Bar

First—and most important—place the bar so it's clear of the other serving tables. You don't want to end up with a huge cluster of people. Some opt to make the kitchen the bar area, but that can be complicated when you're juggling holiday cooking at the same time. If you have the space, it's a better idea to dedicate a table to drinks.

Other tips:

● *Drape the bar top with festive colors,* perhaps a tartan-print or red tablecloth, and add a small vase with holly branches or a potted poinsettia.

● *Offer a specialty cocktail,* which makes for an easy choice for the undecided— and adds a festive air. Try the Cranberry Vodka Spritzer or the Raspberry Moscow Mule (see "Beverages," page 120); put it in a punch bowl, and let people serve themselves. Also include a nonalcoholic punch for nondrinkers and kids.

● *Stock plenty of ice.* Don't rely on your own ice maker; buy bags of commercial cubes. They're easier, and always clearer and prettier.

● *Open several wine bottles* to start things off, and set out at least two corkscrews. To keep whites cold, make a tub of salted ice water (one cup of salt per gallon), which chills much more quickly than ice water alone. Keep a few bar cloths nearby to wipe off drippy bottles.

● *Prep garnishes in advance:* lemon and lime wedges and twists, Maraschino cherries, orange peels, and cocktail olives and onions.

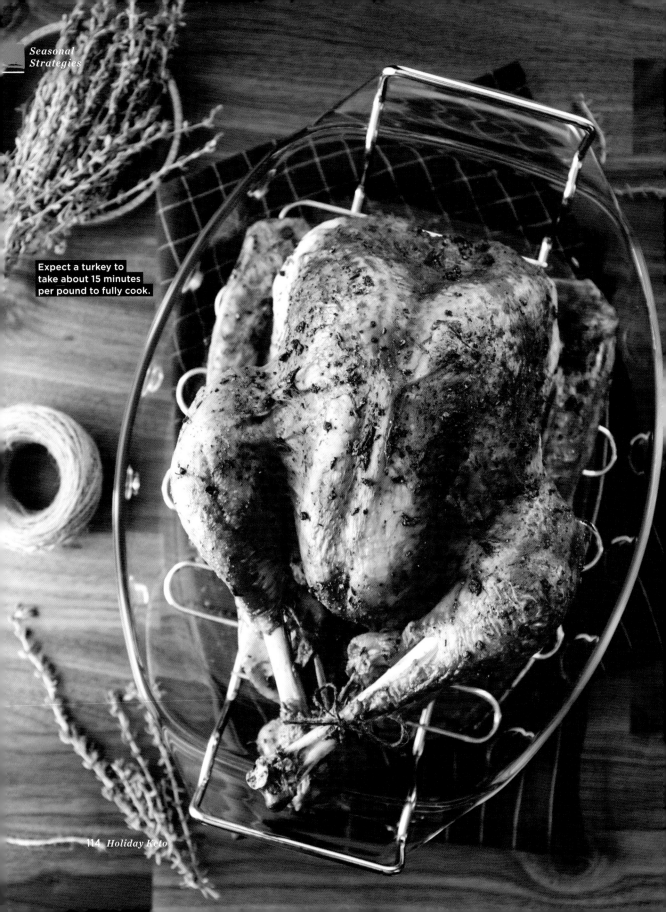

Expect a turkey to take about 15 minutes per pound to fully cook.

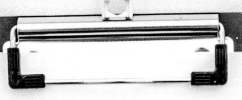

Holiday Dinner Timeline

Big holiday feasts like Thanksgiving are tricky—so many dishes, so many expectations! The best way to wrangle the whole thing is to take it one day at a time, starting a week out. You'll end up having a much better time come the big day. Here's the countdown:

One Week Before

- **Go through your** recipes and make two shopping lists—one for nonperishables like baking supplies and canned goods, and the other for fresh foods that you'll pick up closer to the day of the party. Then go shopping for your first list; that way, your second round at the grocery store (when stores are packed) will be quicker. Be sure to check your pantry and freezer first for staples you assume you already have—baking powder, salt and pepper—just in case, and also check their expiration dates.

- **Buy the booze** and wine, plus any mixers and condiments you need for cocktails.

- **If soup is on the** menu, make it now and freeze it. Take it out the morning of the feast to defrost.

Five Days Before

- **If you're making** a frozen turkey, take it out of the freezer and put it in the refrigerator to thaw. The standard is one day for every 4 pounds, so five days is good for a 20-pounder.

- **Pull out all your** serving bowls and platters and label them with sticky notes for what you'll use them for. This way, you'll know you have what you need. It also makes it easier to delegate tasks to helpers.

- **Clean out your** fridge, getting rid of those nearly-empty pickle jars and anything past its prime. You'll need the space!

Two Days Before

- **Make the keto** bread or cornbread you'll use for the stuffing. Keep it out on the countertop to get "stale."

- **Prepare any** casseroles, let cool and refrigerate. Then you can just reheat them on the big day.

- **Begin baking** desserts that can be stored in airtight containers, like cookies—pies and cakes will have to wait a day.

- **Do your second** shopping trip, picking up a turkey (if using fresh) or meat, fresh vegetables, dairy and other perishables.

One Day Before

- **Chop and prep** vegetables for salads and side dishes, like Brussels sprouts, and store them in airtight bags in the fridge.

- **Most appetizers** can be made now, like dips, pâté, keto bread twists and hard-boiled eggs to be used for deviled eggs.

- **Sauté ingredients** for the stuffing— the onions, celery, sausage, etc. Cool and store in the fridge, then you'll be able to finish making the stuffing the next day in just a few minutes.

- **Make salad** dressing, if needed.

- **Bake last-minute** desserts, like pies.

- **Set the table,** or prep the buffet with everything: plates, silverware, napkins, utensils, decorations. You'll be glad you did!

Feast Day

- **Cook the turkey** (and finish stuffing) or the other main meat course.

- **Heat up anything** you've made in advance: soups, sides, casseroles. Cook any dishes that couldn't be made ahead, like sautéed Brussels sprouts or green bean bundles.

- **Finish day-of** appetizers, like deviled eggs or hot shrimp cocktail. Assemble salad, if it's on the menu.

Voilà, you're ready!

How Much to Make?

Hosting a party this holiday season? Figuring out the right amount of food to serve is a question that tends to drive home cooks crazy. So how can you make sure there's enough delicious keto-friendly fare on hand to feed a crowd? **Don't worry; the pros have a formula for that. Follow these guidelines to make sure everyone leaves your home feeling jolly and satisfied.**

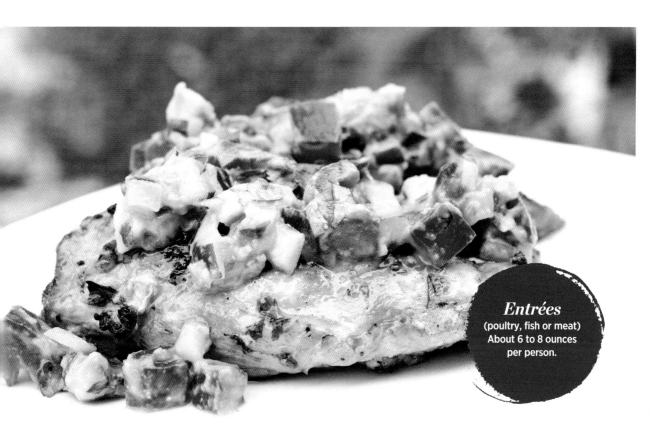

Entrées
(poultry, fish or meat)
About 6 to 8 ounces
per person.

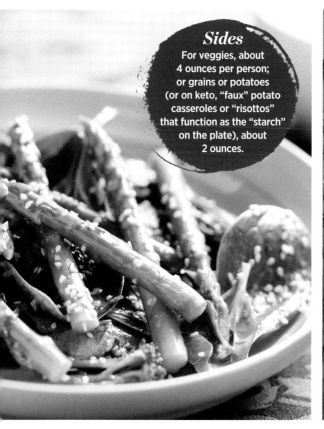

Sides
For veggies, about
4 ounces per person;
or grains or potatoes
(or on keto, "faux" potato
casseroles or "risottos"
that function as the "starch"
on the plate), about
2 ounces.

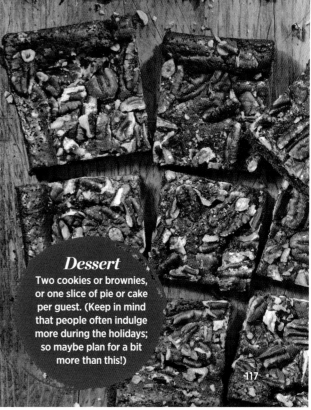

Dessert
Two cookies or brownies,
or one slice of pie or cake
per guest. (Keep in mind
that people often indulge
more during the holidays;
so maybe plan for a bit
more than this!)

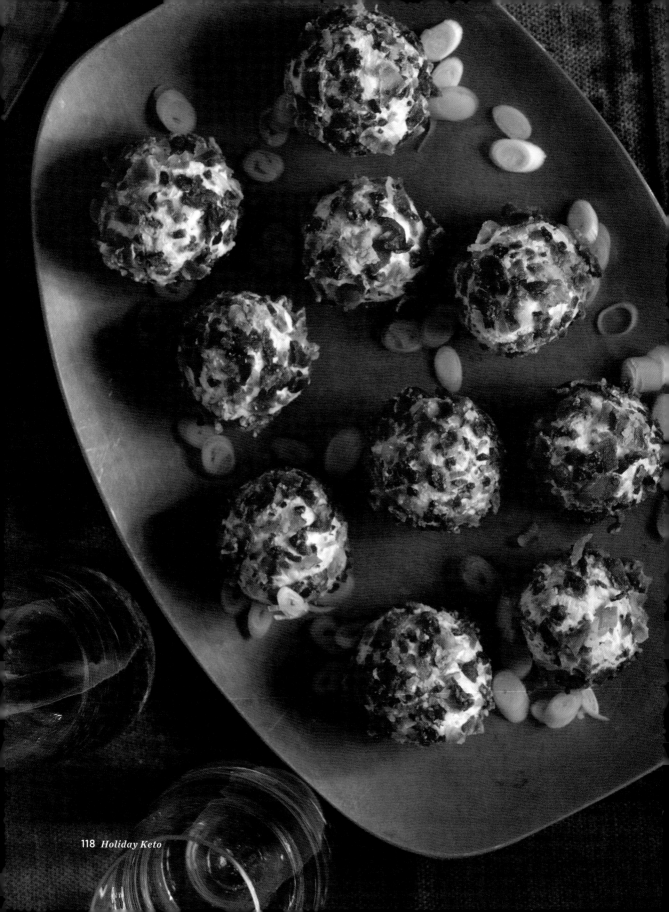

Recipes

THE BEST SEASONAL KETO DISHES FOR YOUR HOLIDAY TABLE.

Beverages

'Tis the season for sipping! Raise a glass with these keto cocktails.

Chocolate Peppermint Cocktail

Chocolate and peppermint are the perfect combination in this delectable, low-carb treat!

PREP 5 minutes
TOTAL 5 minutes
SERVINGS 1

Ingredients

- 2 tablespoons vodka
- 2 teaspoons sugar-free peppermint syrup
- 2 teaspoons sugar-free chocolate syrup
- 2 teaspoons heavy cream
- 1 cup ice cubes
  Garnishes: shaved bittersweet chocolate, crushed sugar-free peppermint candies, whipped cream

Instructions

1 Add all the ingredients in a cocktail shaker. Shake for 30 seconds.
2 Pour into glass and garnish as desired.

NUTRITION INFORMATION (per serving)
Calories: 119; Fat: 5g; Protein: 0g; Carbs: 0.5g; Fiber: 0g; Net Carbs: 0.5g

---

Cranberry Vodka Spritzer

This sweet-tart cocktail is a great-tasting and refreshing beverage—and the garnishes really make it special!

PREP 5 minutes
TOTAL 5 minutes
SERVINGS 1

Ingredients

- ½ cup ice
- 1 tablespoon lime juice
- 2 fluid ounces (2 tablespoons) vodka
- 2 fluid ounces (2 tablespoons) diet cranberry ginger ale
- 2 fluid ounces (2 tablespoons) no-sugar cranberry juice
- 2 fluid ounces (2 tablespoons) cranberry flavored sparkling water
  Garnishes: lime slice, cranberries, orange peel

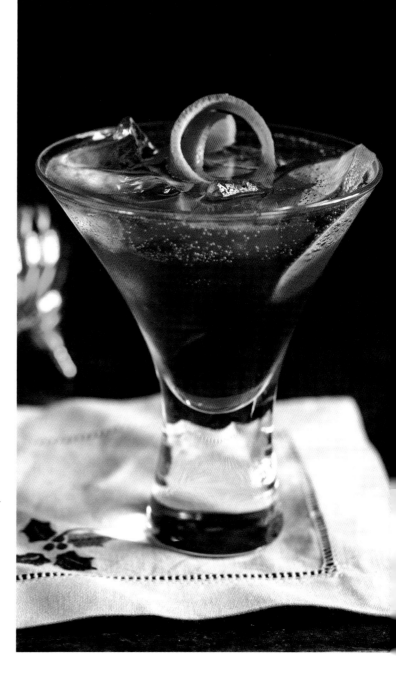

Instructions

1 Place ice cubes in a tall glass.
2 Pour all ingredients into the glass. Stir to combine.
3 Garnish as desired.

NUTRITION INFORMATION (per serving)
Calories: 58; Fat: 0g; Protein: 0g; Carbs: 1g; Fiber: 0g; Net Carbs: 1g

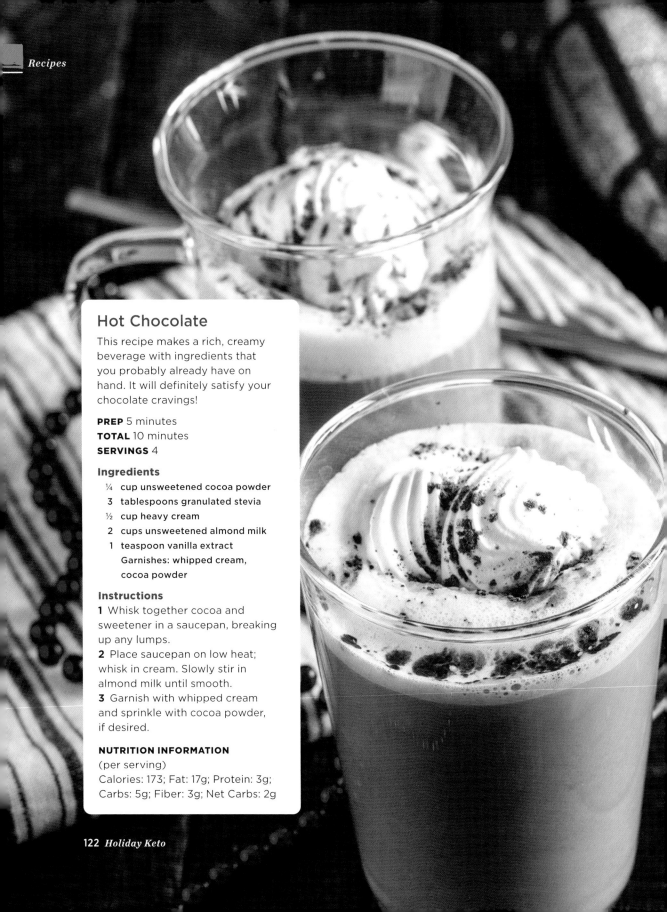

Hot Chocolate

This recipe makes a rich, creamy beverage with ingredients that you probably already have on hand. It will definitely satisfy your chocolate cravings!

PREP 5 minutes
TOTAL 10 minutes
SERVINGS 4

Ingredients

¼ cup unsweetened cocoa powder
3 tablespoons granulated stevia
½ cup heavy cream
2 cups unsweetened almond milk
1 teaspoon vanilla extract
   Garnishes: whipped cream, cocoa powder

Instructions

1 Whisk together cocoa and sweetener in a saucepan, breaking up any lumps.
2 Place saucepan on low heat; whisk in cream. Slowly stir in almond milk until smooth.
3 Garnish with whipped cream and sprinkle with cocoa powder, if desired.

NUTRITION INFORMATION
(per serving)
Calories: 173; Fat: 17g; Protein: 3g; Carbs: 5g; Fiber: 3g; Net Carbs: 2g

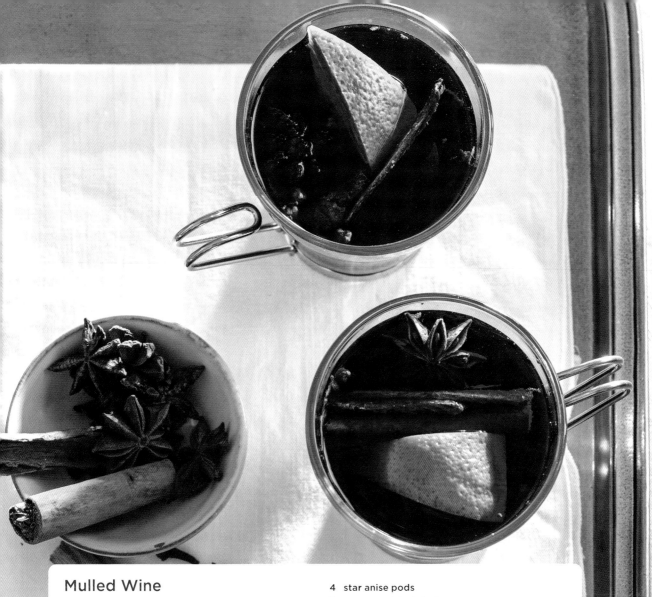

Mulled Wine

Here's a classic recipe that will warm you up on any fall or winter's night! Any dry red wine will work, but use a bottle of Merlot for the best results.

PREP 5 minutes
TOTAL 15 minutes
SERVINGS 6

Ingredients

- 1 (750 ml) bottle of dry red wine
- 1 orange, cut into wedges
- ¼ cup cranberries
- 10 cloves
- 4 cinnamon sticks
- 4 star anise pods
- ⅓ cup granulated stevia
  Garnishes: cinnamon sticks, orange wedges, star anise

Instructions

1 Pour the wine into a saucepan.
2 Add the orange wedges, cranberries, cloves, cinnamon sticks and star anise.
3 Whisk in the sweetener and bring to a simmer over medium heat. Simmer for 15 minutes.
4 Strain into glasses and garnish as desired.

NUTRITION INFORMATION (per serving)
Calories: 122; Fat: 0g; Protein: 0g; Carbs: 4g; Fiber: 0g; Net Carbs: 4g

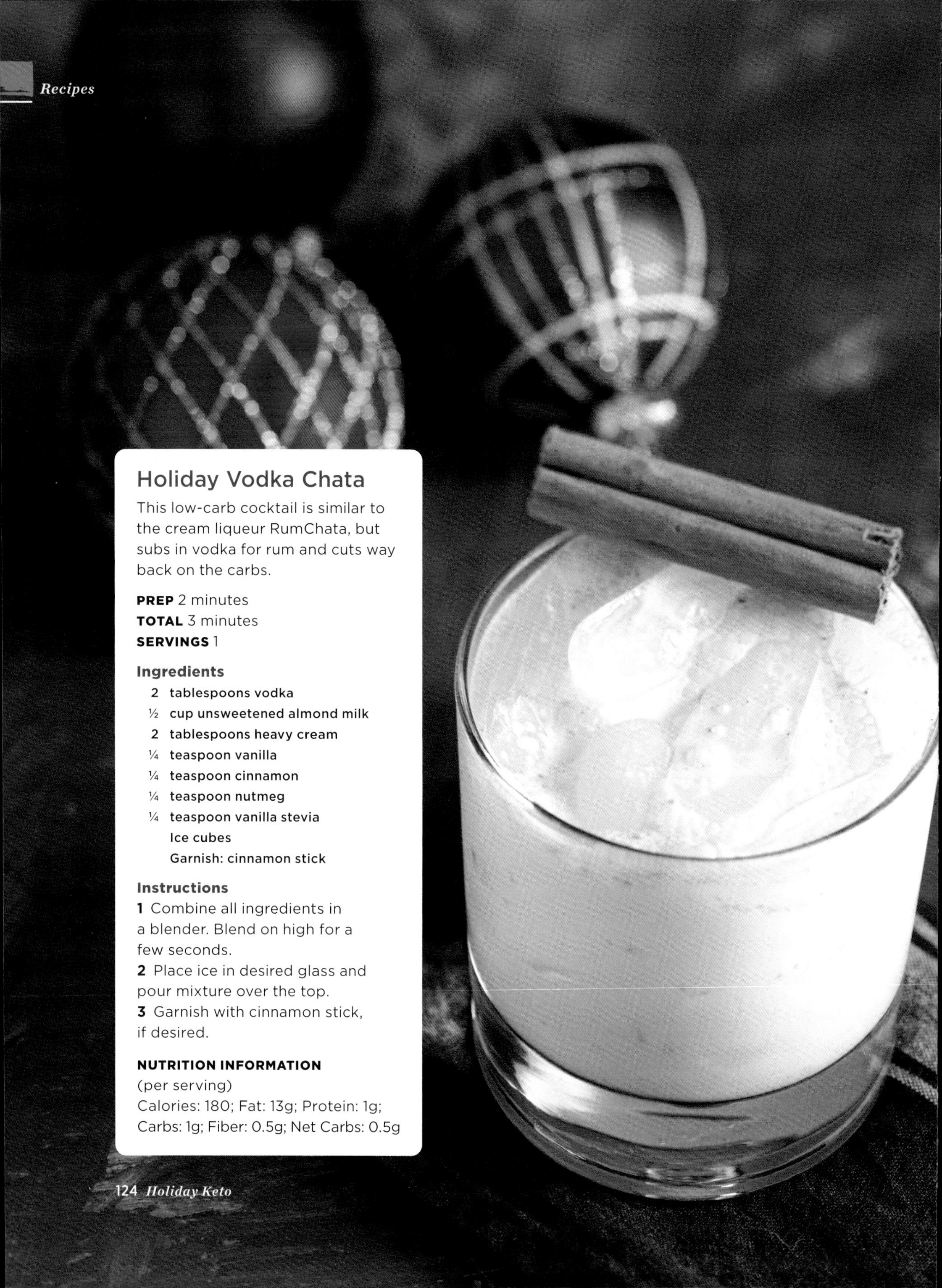

Holiday Vodka Chata

This low-carb cocktail is similar to the cream liqueur RumChata, but subs in vodka for rum and cuts way back on the carbs.

PREP 2 minutes
TOTAL 3 minutes
SERVINGS 1

Ingredients

- 2 tablespoons vodka
- ½ cup unsweetened almond milk
- 2 tablespoons heavy cream
- ¼ teaspoon vanilla
- ¼ teaspoon cinnamon
- ¼ teaspoon nutmeg
- ¼ teaspoon vanilla stevia
  Ice cubes
  Garnish: cinnamon stick

Instructions

1 Combine all ingredients in a blender. Blend on high for a few seconds.
2 Place ice in desired glass and pour mixture over the top.
3 Garnish with cinnamon stick, if desired.

NUTRITION INFORMATION
(per serving)
Calories: 180; Fat: 13g; Protein: 1g; Carbs: 1g; Fiber: 0.5g; Net Carbs: 0.5g

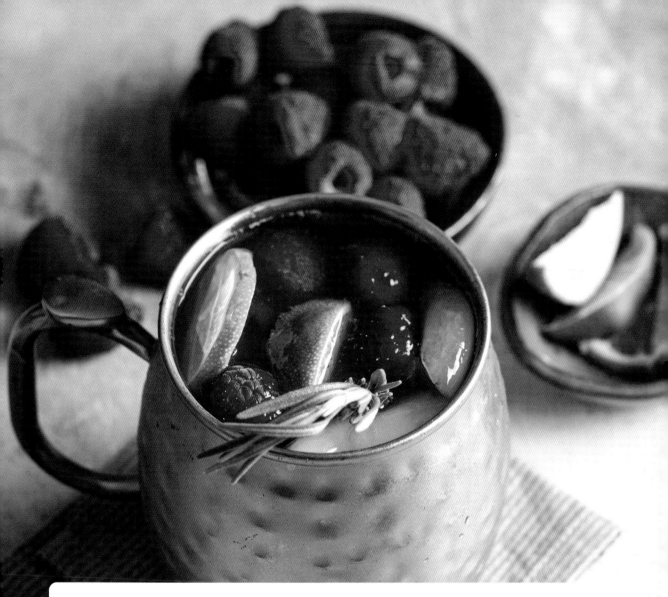

Raspberry Moscow Mule

This delicious and festive cocktail is having a moment, and this version is so delicious you'll never miss the carbs!

PREP 2 minutes
TOTAL 2 minutes
SERVINGS 1

Ingredients

- 3 tablespoons vodka
- 1 (12-ounce) can sugar-free ginger beer (such as Goslings)
- 2 tablespoons diet cranberry juice
- 2 tablespoons lime juice
- 1 cup ice cubes
  Garnishes: raspberries, lime slices and wedges, rosemary sprigs

Instructions

1 Combine vodka, ginger beer, cranberry juice and lime juice in a large glass. Place ice cubes in a copper Moscow mule mug.
2 Pour the mixture over the ice.
3 Garnish as desired.

NUTRITION INFORMATION (per serving)
Calories: 101; Fat: 0g; Protein: 0g; Carbs: 1g; Fiber: 0g; Net Carbs: 1g

Hot Buttered Rum

This sweet and warm drink is super comforting on a chilly night. It's irresistible!

PREP 1 minute
TOTAL 6 minutes
SERVINGS 4

Ingredients

- 2 cups water
- ¼ cup butter
- 1 teaspoon low-carb sweetener (such as monk fruit sweetener)
- 1 teaspoon ground cinnamon
- ½ teaspoon ground nutmeg
- 1 cup dark rum

Instructions

1 Combine water, butter, sweetener, cinnamon and nutmeg in a saucepan and bring to a boil. Reduce heat to a simmer and whisk ingredients.

2 Stir in rum and serve in a glass mug.

NUTRITION INFORMATION
(per serving)
Calories: 243; Fat: 11g; Protein: 0g; Carbs: 0g; Fiber: 0g; Net Carbs: 0g

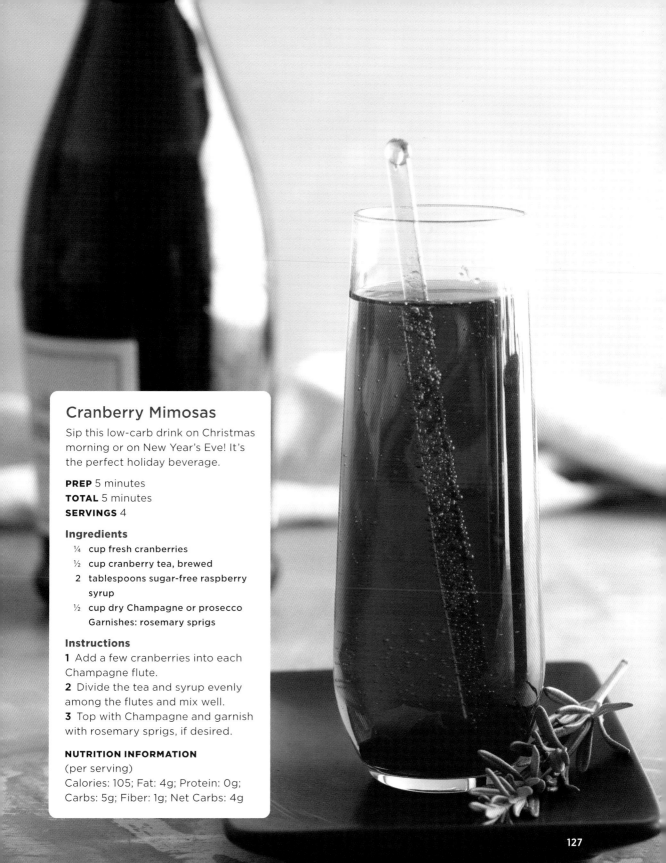

Cranberry Mimosas

Sip this low-carb drink on Christmas morning or on New Year's Eve! It's the perfect holiday beverage.

PREP 5 minutes
TOTAL 5 minutes
SERVINGS 4

Ingredients

- ¼ cup fresh cranberries
- ½ cup cranberry tea, brewed
- 2 tablespoons sugar-free raspberry syrup
- ½ cup dry Champagne or prosecco
  Garnishes: rosemary sprigs

Instructions

1 Add a few cranberries into each Champagne flute.
2 Divide the tea and syrup evenly among the flutes and mix well.
3 Top with Champagne and garnish with rosemary sprigs, if desired.

NUTRITION INFORMATION

(per serving)
Calories: 105; Fat: 4g; Protein: 0g;
Carbs: 5g; Fiber: 1g; Net Carbs: 4g

Eggnog Martini

There's no more fitting cocktail for the holiday season! It's sugar free, but it's wonderfully creamy and decadent.

PREP 5 minutes
TOTAL 20 minutes
SERVINGS 2

Ingredients

- 1 cup heavy cream
- 1 cup unsweetened almond milk
- 2 eggs, beaten
- 2 tablespoons butter
- 2 tablespoons granulated sweetener
- 1 teaspoon vanilla extract
- 1 teaspoon cinnamon
- ½ teaspoon nutmeg
- 2 tablespoons brandy
   Garnishes: whipped cream, fresh grated nutmeg

Instructions

1 In a saucepan over low heat, whisk cream, almond milk, eggs, butter, sweetener, vanilla extract, cinnamon and nutmeg.
2 Cook for 5 minutes. Do not allow to boil. Mixture will thicken slightly.
3 Remove from heat and cool for 15 minutes. Stir in brandy.
4 Pour into 2 martini glasses, garnish with whipped cream and nutmeg, if desired.

NUTRITION INFORMATION
(per serving)
Calories: 125; Fat: 13g; Protein: 1.5g; Carbs: 2g; Fiber: 0g; Net Carbs: 2g

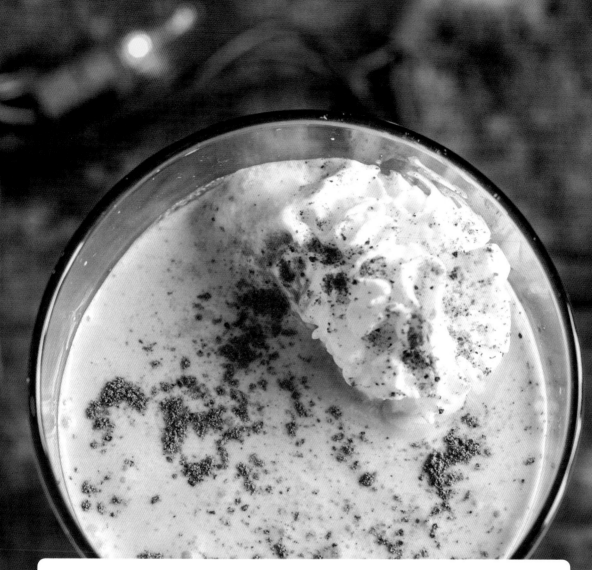

Pumpkin Spice Latte

This recipe tastes like you bought it at a fancy coffee shop! It just doesn't have the carbs and sugar, but it's filled with rich flavor.

PREP 2 minutes
TOTAL 5 minutes
SERVINGS 1

Ingredients

- ¾ cup unsweetened coconut milk
- 2 tablespoons cream
- 2 tablespoons canned pumpkin puree
- 2 teaspoons granulated stevia
- ¼ teaspoon pumpkin pie spice
- ¼ teaspoon vanilla extract
- ½ cup brewed, strong coffee
  Garnishes: whipped cream, pumpkin pie spice

Instructions

1 In a large mug, combine coconut milk, cream, pumpkin, sweetener and pumpkin pie spice.
2 Microwave for 1 minute. Stir in vanilla extract and brewed coffee.
3 Garnish as desired.

NUTRITION INFORMATION (per serving)
Calories: 144; Fat: 13g; Protein: 2g; Carbs: 4g; Fiber: 1g; Net Carbs: 3g

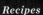

Appetizers

Let's get the party started! Kick off the festivities with keto-approved finger foods.

Spinach Dip With Parmesan Crisps

To make Parmesan crisps, drop heaping tablespoons of grated Parmesan cheese on a silicone baking sheet and press down. Bake for 3 to 5 minutes in a 400°F oven.

PREP 15 minutes
TOTAL 15 minutes
SERVINGS 6

Ingredients

- 1   cup frozen spinach, defrosted, drained and squeezed dry
- 1   cup mayonnaise
- ½   cup sour cream
- 2   tablespoons chopped parsley
- 2   teaspoons lemon juice
- 1   tablespoon dried dill
- 1   teaspoon onion powder
- ½   teaspoon salt
- ½   teaspoon ground black pepper
-     Garnish: parsley leaves
-     Parmesan crisps

Instructions

1 In a large serving bowl, combine all ingredients. Garnish as desired.
2 Serve immediately or refrigerate until ready to serve with Parmesan crisps on the side.

NUTRITION INFORMATION

(per serving, dip only)
Calories: 245; Fat: 20g; Protein: 8g; Carbs: 5g; Fiber: 2g; Net Carbs: 3g

---

Bacon-Wrapped Asparagus

You may want to double the recipe—these are always quick to disappear!

PREP 10 minutes
TOTAL 25 minutes
SERVINGS 6

Ingredients

- 1   tablespoon olive oil
- 6   strips bacon
- 1   ounce cream cheese, softened

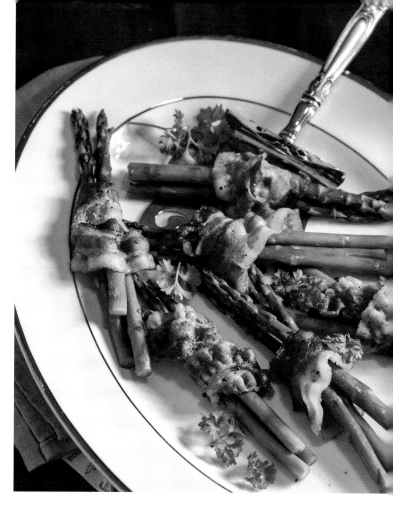

- 18   asparagus spears, trimmed
- 1   teaspoon ground black pepper

Instructions

1 Preheat oven to 450°F. Drizzle a baking sheet with olive oil.
2 Place bacon strips on work surface; spread each with cream cheese.
3 Place 3 asparagus spears across each bacon strip; wrap bacon around spears.
4 Place each bundle seam-side down on prepared baking sheet.
5 Bake for 15 minutes or until crispy, shaking the pan once halfway through cooking time.
6 Sprinkle with pepper; serve hot or at room temperature.

NUTRITION INFORMATION (per serving)

Calories: 185; Fat: 15g; Protein: 5g; Carbs: 3g; Fiber: 1g; Net Carbs: 2g

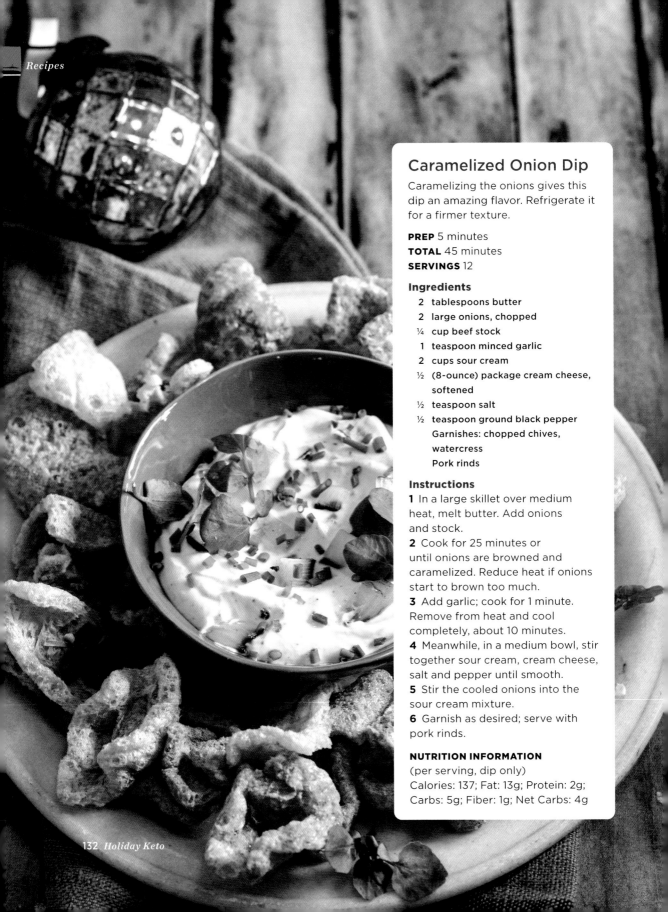

Caramelized Onion Dip

Caramelizing the onions gives this dip an amazing flavor. Refrigerate it for a firmer texture.

PREP 5 minutes
TOTAL 45 minutes
SERVINGS 12

Ingredients

- 2 tablespoons butter
- 2 large onions, chopped
- ¼ cup beef stock
- 1 teaspoon minced garlic
- 2 cups sour cream
- ½ (8-ounce) package cream cheese, softened
- ½ teaspoon salt
- ½ teaspoon ground black pepper
  Garnishes: chopped chives, watercress
  Pork rinds

Instructions

1 In a large skillet over medium heat, melt butter. Add onions and stock.
2 Cook for 25 minutes or until onions are browned and caramelized. Reduce heat if onions start to brown too much.
3 Add garlic; cook for 1 minute. Remove from heat and cool completely, about 10 minutes.
4 Meanwhile, in a medium bowl, stir together sour cream, cream cheese, salt and pepper until smooth.
5 Stir the cooled onions into the sour cream mixture.
6 Garnish as desired; serve with pork rinds.

NUTRITION INFORMATION

(per serving, dip only)
Calories: 137; Fat: 13g; Protein: 2g; Carbs: 5g; Fiber: 1g; Net Carbs: 4g

Spicy Pimento Cheese With Pecans

Called the "caviar of the South," pimento cheese doubles as a dip and a spread. Or try it on top of a burger for a hearty meal.

PREP 10 minutes
TOTAL 10 minutes
SERVINGS 12

Ingredients

- 1 cup mayonnaise
- 4 ounces cream cheese, softened
- 1 (8-ounce) block sharp cheddar, shredded
- 1 (8-ounce) block extra-sharp cheddar cheese, shredded
- 1 teaspoon minced garlic
- 1 (4-ounce) jar pimentos, drained
- ½ teaspoon salt
- ¼ teaspoon cayenne pepper
- ½ cup salted pecans, chopped
  Garnish: chopped pecans
  Keto-friendly crackers and/or crudités
  (cucumber slices, baby red bell peppers)

Instructions

1 In the bowl of a food processor, mix together mayonnaise and cream cheese until they are well combined.

2 Transfer mixture to a large serving bowl; stir in shredded cheeses, garlic, pimentos, salt, cayenne pepper and chopped salted pecans. Garnish as desired.

3 Serve immediately with keto crackers and/or crudités, or cover and refrigerate cheese for up to 5 days.

NUTRITION INFORMATION
(per serving, cheese only)
Calories: 217; Fat: 19g; Protein: 8g; Carbs: 1g; Fiber: 0g; Net Carbs: 1g

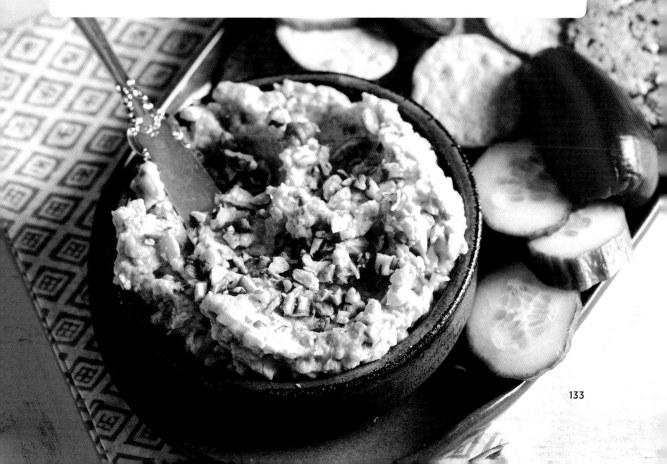

Shrimp With Spicy Remoulade

This creamy New Orleans-style remoulade makes a tasty change from traditional cocktail sauce.

PREP 10 minutes
TOTAL 10 minutes + 2 hours inactive
SERVINGS 8

Ingredients

- 1   cup mayonnaise
- ¼   cup Creole mustard
- 1   tablespoon paprika
- 2   teaspoons Creole seasoning
- 1   tablespoon horseradish
- 1   teaspoon garlic powder
- ½   teaspoon cayenne pepper
- ½   teaspoon Worcestershire sauce
- 1   pound large tail-on shrimp, peeled, deveined and cooked
  Garnish: parsley leaves

Instructions

1 In a medium bowl, combine mayonnaise, mustard, paprika, Creole seasoning, horseradish, garlic powder, cayenne pepper and Worcestershire sauce. Cover and refrigerate for 2 hours.

2 Transfer remoulade to a footed dish. Place dish in center of serving platter; arrange shrimp around dish. Garnish as desired.

NUTRITION INFORMATION
(per serving)
Calories: 225; Fat: 12g; Protein: 15g; Carbs: 4g; Fiber: 0.5g; Net Carbs: 3.5g

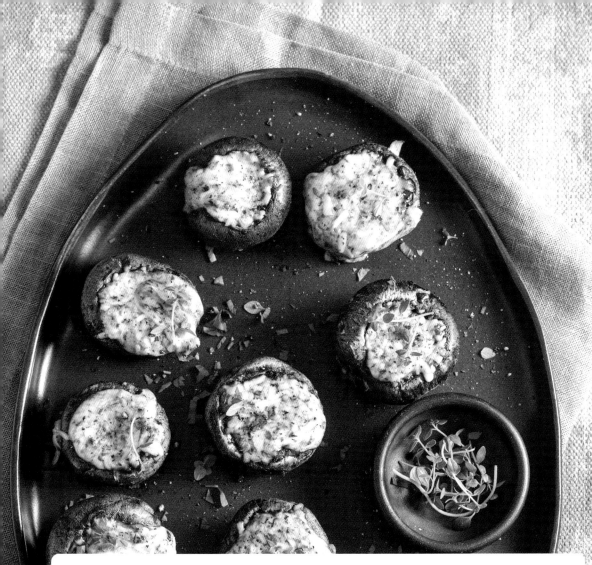

Italian Sausage Stuffed Mushrooms

Spicy sausage and thyme give these mushrooms loads of flavor. If you don't love spicy, swap the hot sausage for sweet.

PREP 10 minutes
TOTAL 20 minutes
SERVINGS 16

Ingredients

- ½ pound hot Italian sausage, cooked and crumbled
- 4 ounces cream cheese, softened
- ½ cup shredded mozzarella
- ½ teaspoon salt
- ½ teaspoon ground black pepper
- 16 small portobello mushroom caps, cleaned, gills removed
  Garnishes: thyme sprigs, cracked black pepper

Instructions

1 Preheat oven to 350°F.
2 In a bowl, combine sausage, cream cheese, mozzarella, salt and pepper.
3 Spoon sausage mixture into mushroom caps; place stuffing side up on baking sheet. Bake for 10 minutes.
4 Garnish as desired; serve immediately.

NUTRITION INFORMATION (per serving)
Calories: 375; Fat: 35g; Protein: 18g; Carbs: 9g; Fiber: 2g; Net Carbs: 7g

Mini Cheese Truffles

These are not only delicious, they're super quick to put together and travel extremely well, so they're a perfect appetizer to take to a party as a guest!

PREP 10 minutes
TOTAL 10 minutes
SERVINGS 10 (3 truffles per serving)

Ingredients

- 1 (8-ounce) block sharp cheddar cheese, shredded
- 1 (8-ounce) block cream cheese, softened
- ¼ cup chopped green onions
- ½ teaspoon ground black pepper
- 2 cups cooked bacon, chopped or crumbled
  Garnish: minced green onions

Instructions

1 In a bowl, combine cheddar cheese, cream cheese, chopped green onions and pepper.
2 Use a small cookie scoop to form mixture into tablespoon-size balls.
3 Roll balls in bacon; garnish platter with minced green onions.
4 Serve immediately, or cover and refrigerate until ready to serve.

NUTRITION INFORMATION (per serving)
Calories: 192; Fat: 12g; Protein: 7g; Carbs: 1g; Fiber: 0g; Net Carbs: 1g

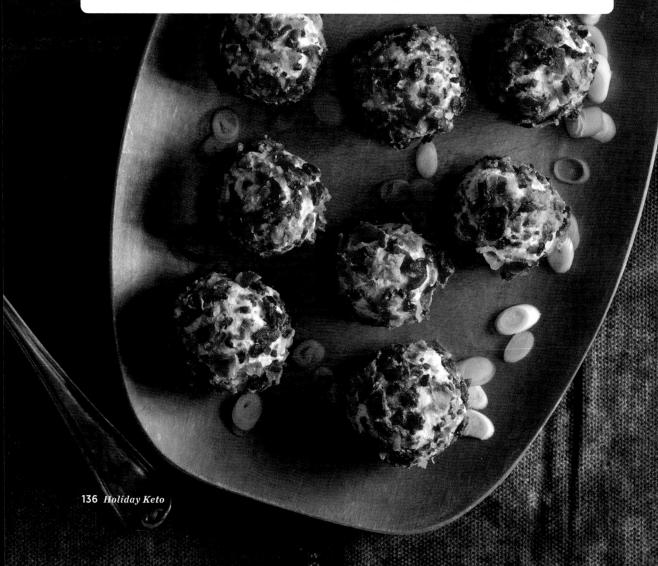

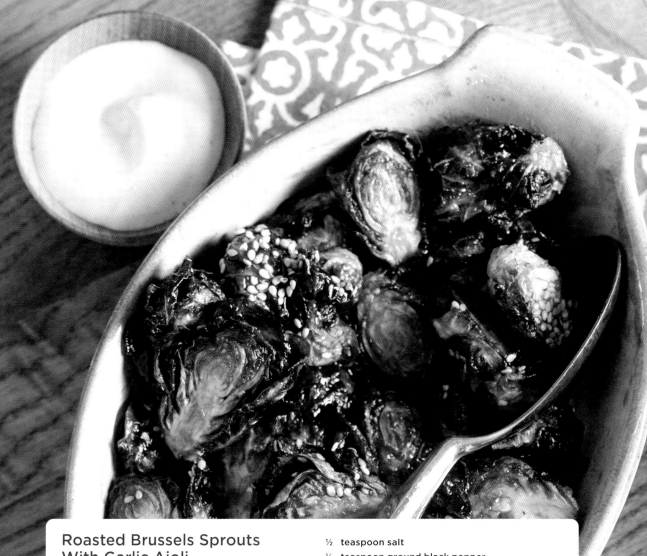

Roasted Brussels Sprouts With Garlic Aioli

You may even convert some sprouts-haters with this addictive dish. Store-bought aioli cuts your prep time significantly.

PREP 10 minutes
TOTAL 35 minutes
SERVINGS 4

Ingredients

- 1 pound fresh Brussels sprouts, trimmed and halved
- 2 tablespoons olive oil
- 2 teaspoons gluten-free soy sauce
- 1 teaspoon minced garlic
- 2 teaspoons lemon juice
- ½ teaspoon salt
- ½ teaspoon ground black pepper
   Garlic aioli

Instructions

1 Preheat oven to 400°F.
2 In a large bowl, toss together sprouts, olive oil, soy sauce, garlic, lemon juice, salt and pepper. On a large baking sheet, arrange sprouts in a single layer.
3 Bake for 20 to 25 minutes, or until sprouts are golden brown.
4 Serve garlic aioli on the side for dipping.

NUTRITION INFORMATION
(per serving, sprouts only)
Calories: 172; Fat: 14g; Protein: 2g; Carbs: 10g; Fiber: 2g; Net Carbs: 8g

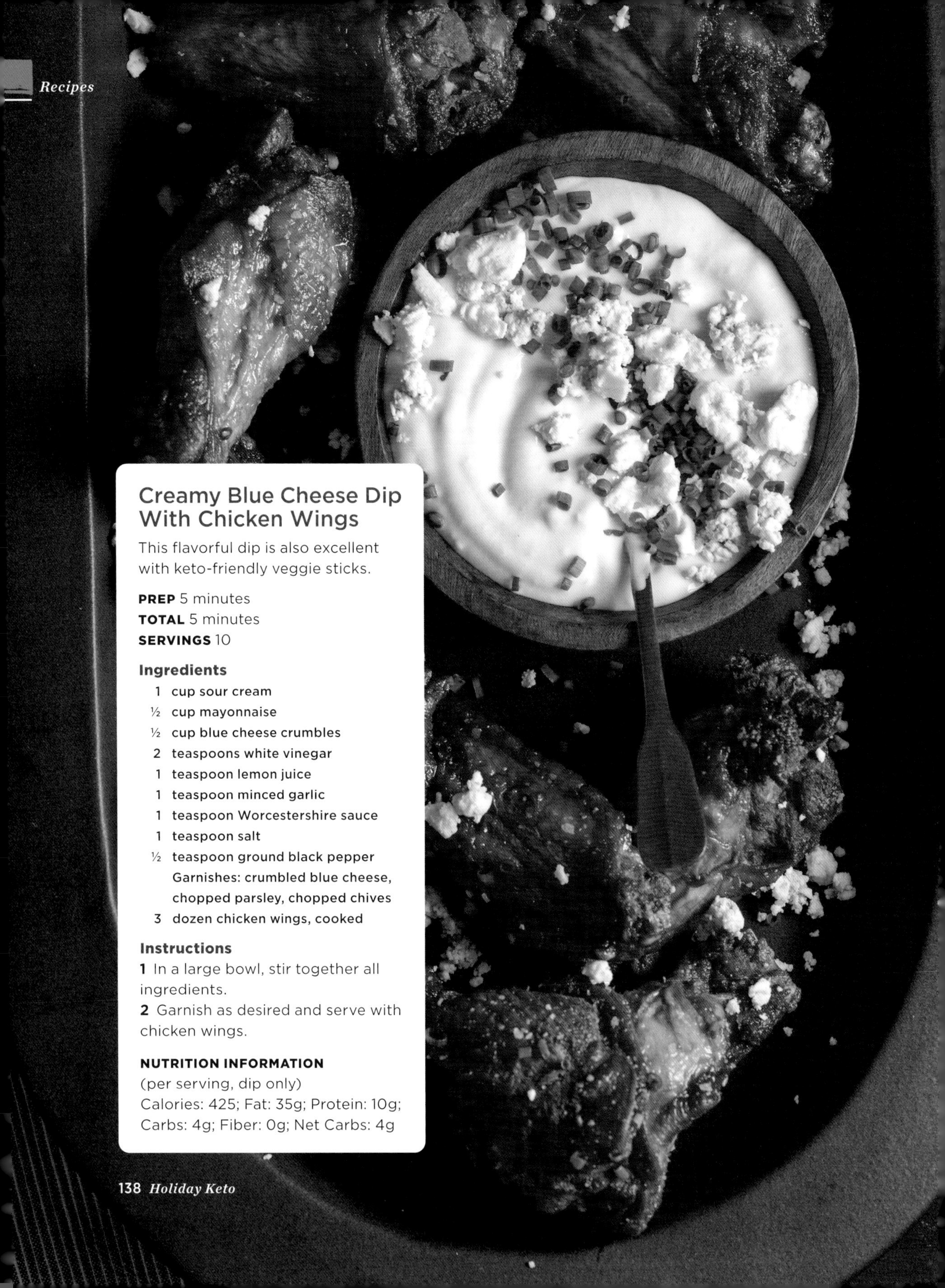

Creamy Blue Cheese Dip With Chicken Wings

This flavorful dip is also excellent with keto-friendly veggie sticks.

PREP 5 minutes
TOTAL 5 minutes
SERVINGS 10

Ingredients

- 1 cup sour cream
- ½ cup mayonnaise
- ½ cup blue cheese crumbles
- 2 teaspoons white vinegar
- 1 teaspoon lemon juice
- 1 teaspoon minced garlic
- 1 teaspoon Worcestershire sauce
- 1 teaspoon salt
- ½ teaspoon ground black pepper
  Garnishes: crumbled blue cheese, chopped parsley, chopped chives
- 3 dozen chicken wings, cooked

Instructions

1 In a large bowl, stir together all ingredients.
2 Garnish as desired and serve with chicken wings.

NUTRITION INFORMATION
(per serving, dip only)
Calories: 425; Fat: 35g; Protein: 10g; Carbs: 4g; Fiber: 0g; Net Carbs: 4g

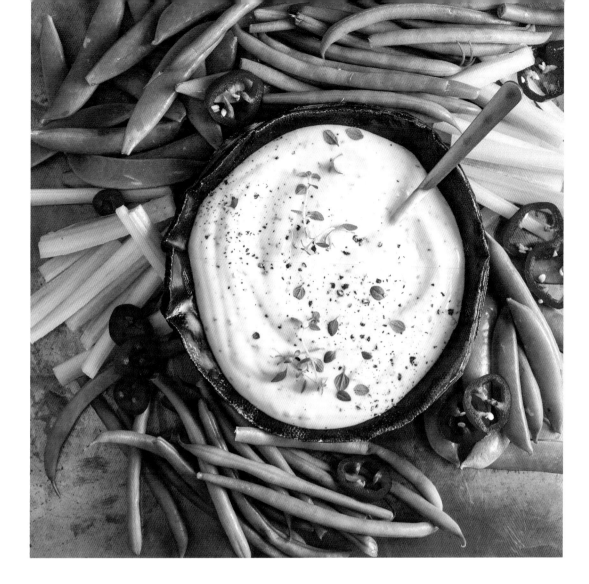

Homemade Ranch Dip
With Assorted Vegetables

Make an extra batch of this ranch to use as a super-creamy salad dressing. Assorted crudités provide some crunch with every bite.

PREP 5 minutes
TOTAL 5 minutes + 2 hours inactive
SERVINGS 10

Ingredients

- ½ cup mayonnaise
- ½ cup sour cream
- 2 tablespoons white vinegar
- 2 tablespoons chopped dill
- 1 tablespoon chopped parsley
- 1 teaspoon chopped chives
- 1 teaspoon minced garlic
- 1 teaspoon onion powder
- 1 teaspoon salt
- ½ teaspoon ground black pepper
  Garnishes: thyme sprigs, cracked black pepper
  Assorted crudités: sugar snap peas, haricots verts, celery sticks, sliced Fresno peppers

Instructions

1 In a serving bowl, mix all ingredients. Cover and refrigerate for 2 hours.
2 Garnish as desired; serve with crudités.

NUTRITION INFORMATION (per serving, dip only)
Calories: 241; Fat: 20g; Protein: 1g; Carbs: 1g; Fiber: 0g; Net Carbs: 1g

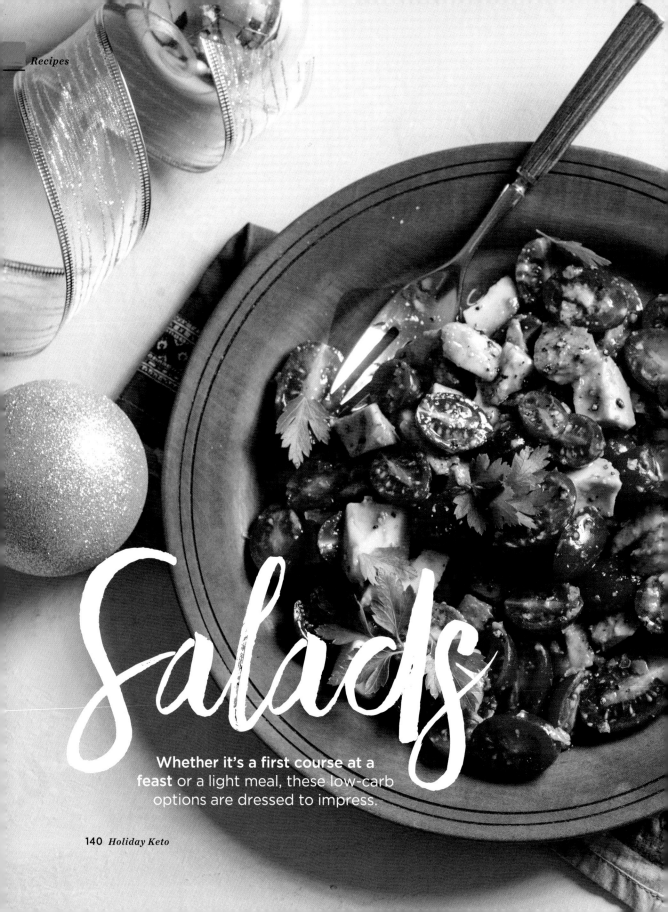

Salads

Whether it's a first course at a feast or a light meal, these low-carb options are dressed to impress.

Holiday Salad With Tomatoes and Avocado

Toss some bacon crumbles on this salad right before serving for a tasty variation.

PREP 10 minutes
TOTAL 10 minutes
SERVINGS 4

Ingredients

2 cups grape tomatoes, halved
2 avocados, cubed
½ teaspoon sea salt
½ teaspoon ground black pepper
1 tablespoon lime juice
Garnishes: parsley sprigs, olive oil drizzle

Instructions

Add all ingredients to a bowl and toss together. Garnish as desired.

NUTRITION INFORMATION (per serving)
Calories: 177; Fat: 14.5g; Protein: 3g; Carbs: 12g; Fiber: 8g; Net Carbs: 4g

---

Spinach Salad With Eggs and Bacon

This classic salad is great for lunch or as a starter for a holiday dinner.

PREP 20 minutes
TOTAL 20 minutes
SERVINGS 4

Ingredients

3 tablespoons olive oil
1 tablespoon white wine vinegar
½ teaspoon garlic paste
¼ teaspoon salt
¼ teaspoon ground black pepper
4 cups baby spinach
⅓ cup cooked, crumbled bacon
4 hard-boiled eggs, sliced

Instructions

1 In a small bowl, whisk together olive oil, vinegar, garlic paste, salt and pepper.
2 In a large bowl, toss spinach and bacon.
3 Pour dressing over salad; top with sliced hard-boiled eggs.

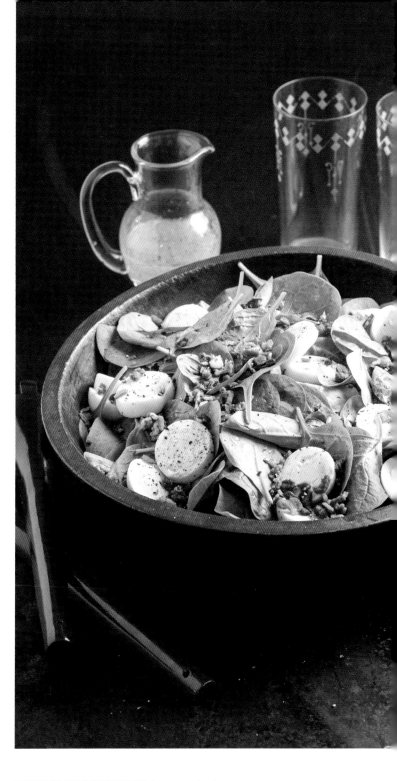

NUTRITION INFORMATION (per serving)
Calories: 212; Fat: 18g; Protein: 9.5g; Carbs: 1g; Fiber: 1g; Net Carbs: 0g

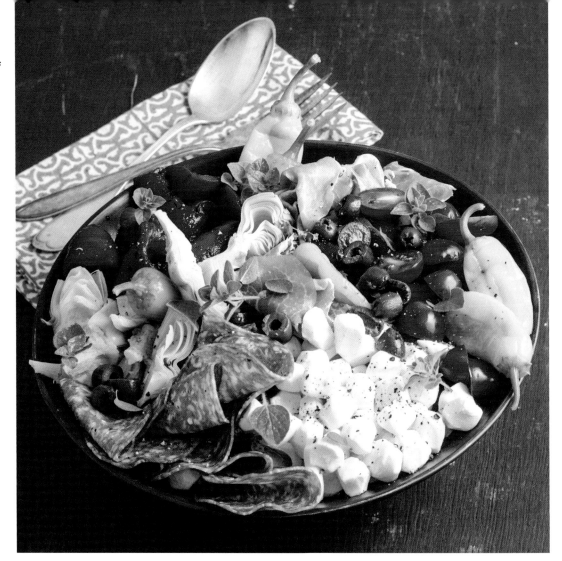

Italian Antipasto Salad

Make this dish up to two days ahead. This dressing is outrageous—try it on any salad!

PREP 10 minutes
TOTAL 10 minutes
SERVINGS 8

Ingredients

- ¼ cup olive oil
- 1 tablespoon red wine vinegar
- ½ teaspoon sea salt
- ¼ teaspoon ground black pepper
- ¼ cup chopped basil
- 1 (4-ounce) package sliced salami
- 1 (3-ounce) container fresh mozzarella balls, drained
- 1 (6-ounce) package sliced prosciutto
- 2 cups grape tomatoes, halved
- 1 cup pepperoncini peppers
- 1 cup roasted red peppers
- 1 (14-ounce) can artichoke hearts, drained and halved
- ½ cup kalamata olives, pitted and halved
  Garnish: basil leaves

Instructions

1 In a large bowl, whisk together oil, vinegar, salt, pepper and chopped basil.
2 Add all remaining ingredients to serving bowl; toss to combine. Garnish as desired.

NUTRITION INFORMATION (per serving)
Calories: 345; Fat: 30g; Protein: 14g; Carbs: 3g; Fiber: 1g; Net Carbs: 2g

Arugula Salad With Feta and Cranberries

This light and flavorful salad pairs well with roasted lamb or chicken.

PREP 10 minutes
TOTAL 10 minutes
SERVINGS 4

Ingredients

- 4 cups arugula
- ⅓ cup crumbled feta cheese
- 1 tablespoon reduced-sugar dried cranberries
- 2 tablespoons olive oil
- 1 tablespoon balsamic vinegar
- ½ teaspoon sea salt
- ¼ teaspoon ground black pepper

Instructions

1 Place arugula in a serving bowl; top with feta and cranberries.

2 To make dressing, in a small bowl, combine olive oil, vinegar, salt and pepper. Pour over salad, toss and serve.

NUTRITION INFORMATION (per serving)
Calories: 97; Fat: 7g; Protein: 3g; Carbs: 7g; Fiber: 1g; Net Carbs: 6g

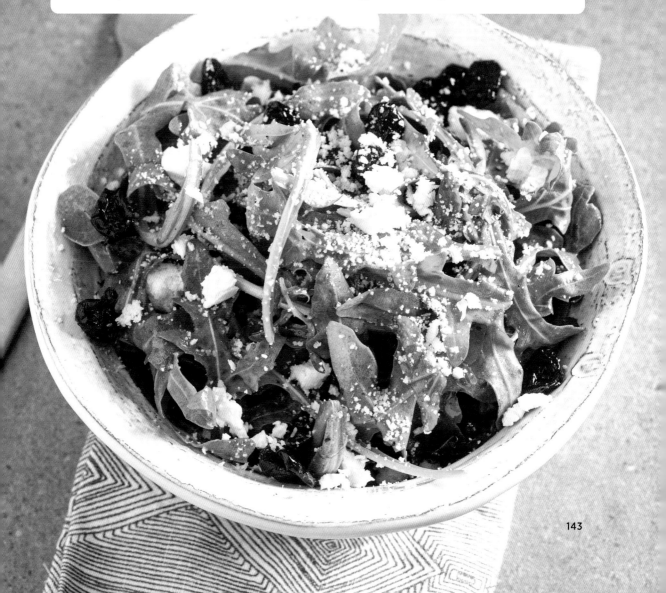

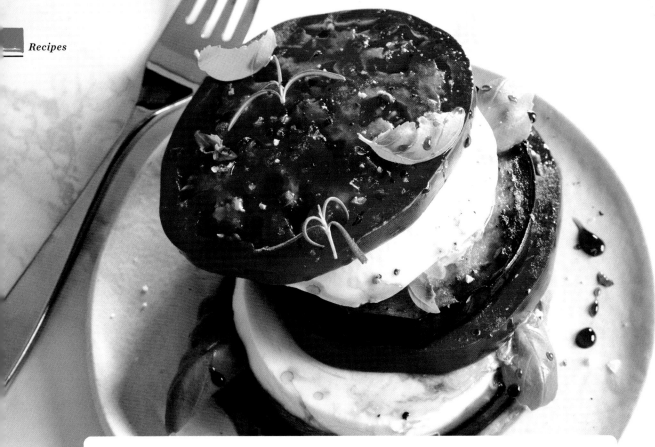

Eggplant and Tomato Stacks With Rosemary

Even non-ketoers will love this twist on the classic Caprese salad.

PREP 10 minutes
TOTAL 20 minutes
SERVINGS 4

Ingredients

- ½ cup plus 2 tablespoons extra-virgin olive oil, divided
- 2 tablespoons balsamic vinegar
- 1 teaspoon minced garlic
- 1 teaspoon minced rosemary
- ½ teaspoon salt
- ½ teaspoon ground black pepper
- 1 (1-pound) eggplant, cut into eight ½-inch-thick slices
- 8 basil leaves
- 1 (8-ounce) block fresh mozzarella, cut into 8 slices
- 4 large tomatoes, cut into eight ¼-inch-thick slices
- Garnishes: rosemary sprigs, basil leaves, balsamic glaze

Instructions

1 To make dressing, in a blender or food processor, blend ½ cup olive oil, vinegar, garlic, rosemary, salt and pepper until smooth. Set dressing aside.
2 In a skillet over medium-high heat, heat remaining 2 tablespoons olive oil.
3 Fry eggplant slices until golden, about 2 minutes per side.
4 Place an eggplant slice in the center of each serving plate; top each with a basil leaf, a mozzarella slice and a tomato slice. Repeat layers once.
5 Spoon dressing over the top of each stack; garnish as desired.

NUTRITION INFORMATION (per serving)
Calories: 487; Fat: 43g; Protein: 14g; Carbs: 13g; Fiber: 8g; Net Carbs: 5g

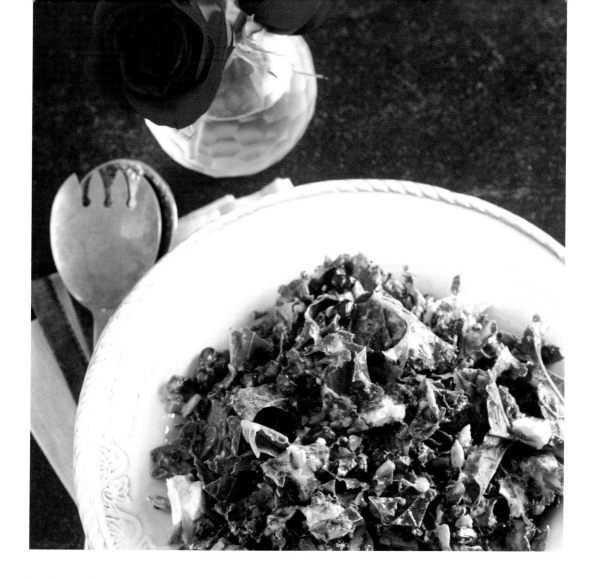

Kale Salad With Goat Cheese and Pomegranate Seeds

This red-and-green salad makes an attractive addition to a holiday table.

PREP 15 minutes
TOTAL 15 minutes
SERVINGS 4

Ingredients

- ¼ cup olive oil
- 3 tablespoons balsamic vinegar
- ¾ teaspoon Dijon mustard
- ⅔ teaspoon minced garlic
- ½ teaspoon sea salt, divided
- 2 teaspoons chopped parsley
- 1½ bunches kale, ribs and stems removed
- 3 ounces goat cheese, crumbled
- ⅔ cup pomegranate seeds
- ¼ cup toasted sunflower seeds
- ¼ teaspoon ground black pepper

Instructions

1 To make dressing, in a blender, mix olive oil, vinegar, mustard, garlic, ¼ teaspoon salt and parsley until smooth.
2 In a large serving bowl, add kale. Top with goat cheese, pomegranate seeds, sunflower seeds, remaining ¼ teaspoon salt and pepper.
3 Pour dressing over salad; serve.

NUTRITION INFORMATION (per serving)
Calories: 285; Fat: 20g; Protein: 11g; Carbs: 10g; Fiber: 3g; Net Carbs: 7g

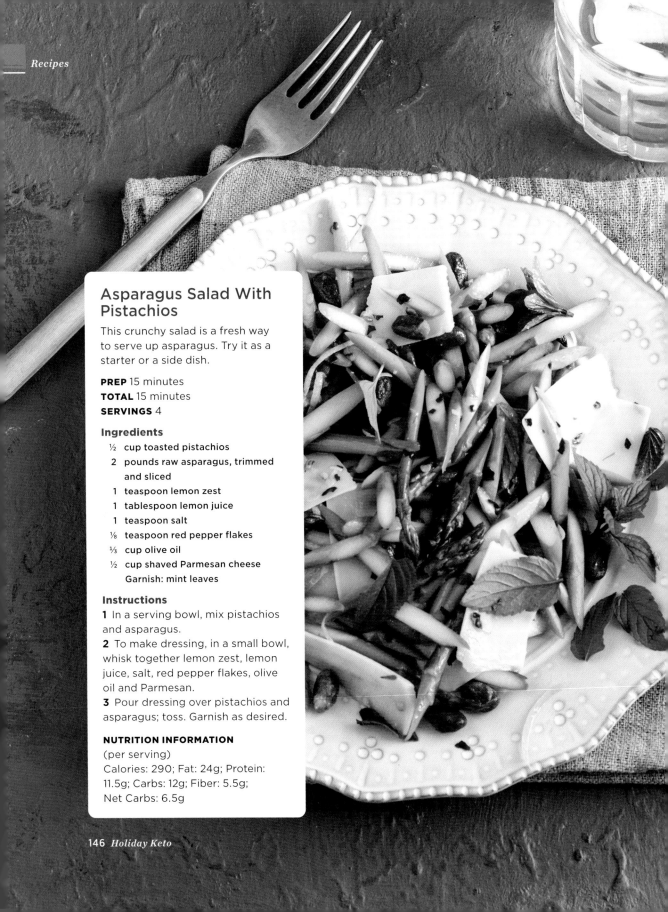

Asparagus Salad With Pistachios

This crunchy salad is a fresh way to serve up asparagus. Try it as a starter or a side dish.

PREP 15 minutes
TOTAL 15 minutes
SERVINGS 4

Ingredients

- ½ cup toasted pistachios
- 2 pounds raw asparagus, trimmed and sliced
- 1 teaspoon lemon zest
- 1 tablespoon lemon juice
- 1 teaspoon salt
- ⅛ teaspoon red pepper flakes
- ⅓ cup olive oil
- ½ cup shaved Parmesan cheese
  Garnish: mint leaves

Instructions

1 In a serving bowl, mix pistachios and asparagus.
2 To make dressing, in a small bowl, whisk together lemon zest, lemon juice, salt, red pepper flakes, olive oil and Parmesan.
3 Pour dressing over pistachios and asparagus; toss. Garnish as desired.

NUTRITION INFORMATION

(per serving)
Calories: 290; Fat: 24g; Protein: 11.5g; Carbs: 12g; Fiber: 5.5g; Net Carbs: 6.5g

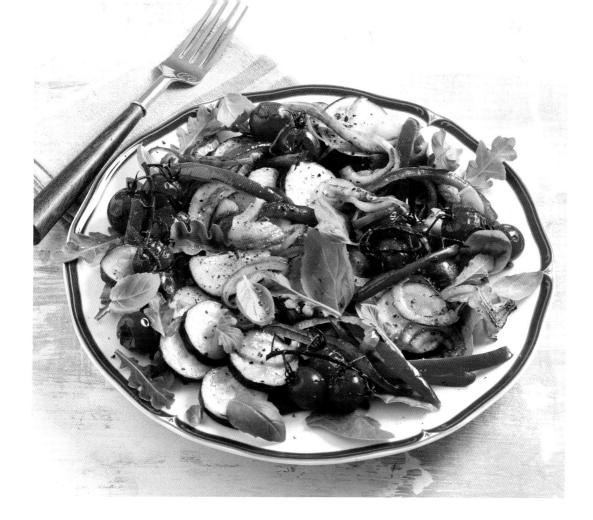

Roasted Vegetable Salad

When you're craving the flavors of summer, try this easy-to-assemble salad. Roasting the vegetables enhances their flavor, so they taste as good as if you'd just picked them up at the farmstand. Regular cherry tomatoes can be substituted for the on-the-vine type.

PREP 15 minutes
TOTAL 40 minutes
SERVINGS 4

Ingredients

1   zucchini, sliced
1   cup cherry tomatoes on the vine
1   red bell pepper, sliced
1   red onion, sliced
1   head garlic, halved
¼   cup olive oil
½   teaspoon sea salt
½   teaspoon ground black pepper
1   cup arugula
1   cup baby spinach leaves
    Garnish: basil leaves

Instructions

1 Preheat oven to 400°F.
2 Place zucchini, tomatoes, bell pepper, onion and garlic on a baking sheet.
3 Drizzle vegetables with olive oil; sprinkle with salt and pepper.
4 Roast vegetables for 20 to 25 minutes. Remove from oven; let cool.
5 On a serving platter, arrange arugula and spinach; top with roasted vegetables.
6 Drizzle with additional olive oil and garnish as desired.

NUTRITION INFORMATION (per serving)
Calories: 113; Fat: 7g; Protein: 2g; Carbs: 11g; Fiber: 4g; Net Carbs: 7g

Soups

Warm up on a cool day with hearty fare. It's mmm-mmm good!

Clam Chowder

This five-ingredient soup is ready in just 15 minutes, but it tastes like you cooked all day!

PREP 5 minutes
TOTAL 20 minutes
SERVINGS 6

Ingredients

- 2 (6.5-ounce) cans clams, undrained
- 4 cups cauliflower florets
- 1½ cups almond milk
- 1½ cups chicken broth
- 1 teaspoon sea salt
- ½ teaspoon ground black pepper
- 1 cup coconut cream
  Garnishes: cracked black pepper, parsley leaves

Instructions

1 In a Dutch oven, combine all ingredients except for the coconut cream.
2 Bring to a boil. Reduce heat and simmer for 10 to 15 minutes or until the cauliflower is tender.
3 Stir in coconut cream. Serve soup and garnish as desired.

NUTRITION INFORMATION (per serving)
Calories: 228; Fat: 16g; Protein: 12g; Carbs: 11g; Fiber: 4g; Net Carbs: 7g

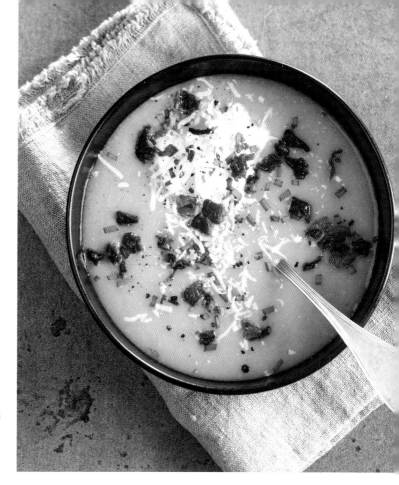

Bacon and Cauliflower Soup

This soup is smooth, creamy and wonderfully delicious.

PREP 15 minutes
TOTAL 40 minutes
SERVINGS 6

Ingredients

- 1 tablespoon butter
- 1 teaspoon minced garlic
- 1½ pounds cauliflower florets
- 2 cups chicken stock
- 1½ cups heavy cream
- 1 teaspoon salt
- 1 teaspoon ground black pepper
- 4 strips bacon, cooked and crumbled
- ⅔ cup grated Parmesan cheese
  Garnishes: Parmesan cheese, chopped chives, sour cream, crumbled bacon

Instructions

1 In a Dutch oven over high heat, sauté butter and garlic for 3 minutes.
2 Add the cauliflower and stir to coat. Cook for 2 minutes.
3 Stir in chicken stock, cream, salt and pepper. Bring to a boil, then reduce heat to a simmer.
4 Cook for 15 minutes, or until the cauliflower is tender.
5 Using an immersion blender, blend the soup into a smooth puree.
6 Stir in the bacon and Parmesan cheese.
7 Serve soup and garnish as desired.

NUTRITION INFORMATION (per serving)
Calories: 345; Fat: 34g; Protein: 15g; Carbs: 8g; Fiber: 3g; Net Carbs: 5g

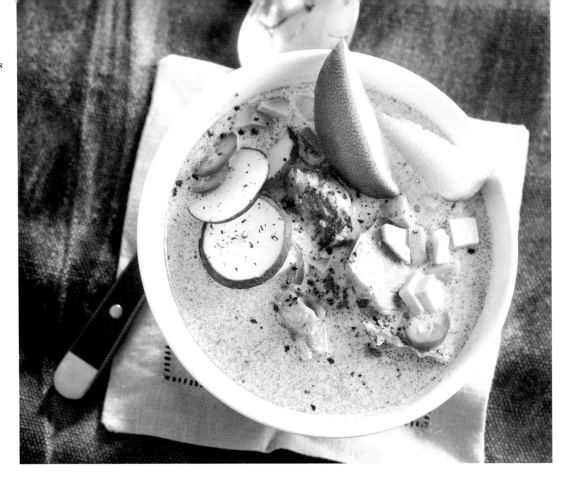

Leftover Turkey Chowder

The one-pot soup is a perfect way to use your leftover holiday bird. Bonus: It's ready in just 20 minutes, and the Mexican seasonings make it a nice change from the usual turkey soups.

PREP 10 minutes
TOTAL 20 minutes
SERVINGS 6

Ingredients

- ¼ cup olive oil
- 1 cup chopped onion
- 1 green bell pepper, chopped
- 2 jalapeños, chopped
- 1 teaspoon minced garlic
- 1 tablespoon taco seasoning
- ½ teaspoon sea salt
- ½ teaspoon ground black pepper
- 1 (4-ounce) can diced green chiles
- 4 cups turkey or chicken broth
- 1 tablespoon lime juice
- 1 cup heavy cream
- 4 ounces cream cheese
- 1 pound leftover chopped or shredded turkey
  Garnishes: chopped avocado, lime wedges, sliced jalapeño peppers, sliced radishes, cracked black pepper

Instructions

1 In a Dutch oven, heat the olive oil over medium high heat.

2 Add onion, bell pepper, jalapeños and garlic. Sauté for 5 minutes.

3 Add the spices and cook 1 minute. Stir in the green chiles and broth. Bring to a simmer, cover and cook for 5 minutes. Stir in lime juice.

4 Remove the lid and stir in the heavy cream and cream cheese. Simmer 3 minutes and whisk to smooth out any lumps.

5 Add the turkey and cook 1 more minute.

6 Serve soup and garnish as desired.

NUTRITION INFORMATION (per serving)
Calories: 334; Fat: 23g; Protein: 30g; Carbs: 8g; Fiber: 2g; Net Carbs: 6g

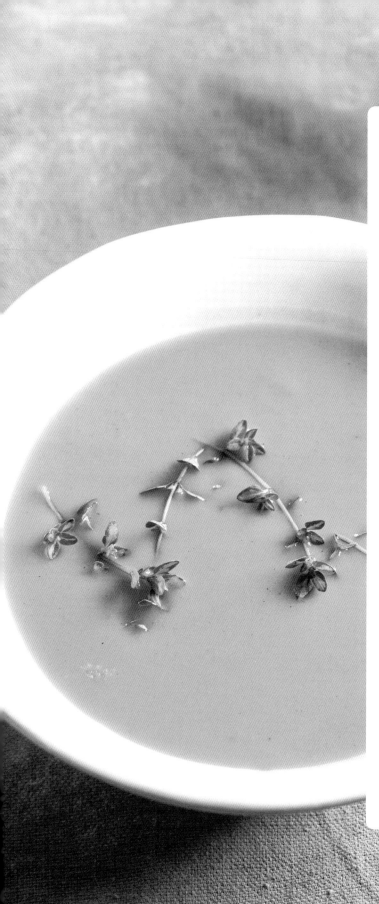

Roasted Butternut Squash Bisque

Dairy-free and nut-free, this creamy soup gets its richness from coconut milk. It makes a sensational first course for a holiday feast.

PREP 10 minutes
TOTAL 1 hour 10 minutes
SERVINGS 8

Ingredients

- 8 cups cubed butternut squash
- 2 tablespoons olive oil, divided
- ½ teaspoon sea salt
- ½ teaspoon ground black pepper
- 2 tablespoons minced garlic
- 2 sprigs fresh thyme
- ½ teaspoon cinnamon
- ⅛ teaspoon nutmeg
- 4 cups chicken broth
- 1 (13.5-ounce) can coconut milk
  Garnish: thyme sprigs

Instructions

1 Preheat oven to 400°F.
2 Line a baking sheet with aluminum foil.
3 Place the cubed squash on the baking sheet and drizzle with 1 tablespoon olive oil. Sprinkle with salt and pepper.
4 Roast for 15 to 20 minutes.
5 In a Dutch oven, add remaining 1 tablespoon olive oil. Stir in garlic, thyme sprigs, cinnamon and nutmeg. Sauté for 1 more minute.
6 Add broth, coconut milk and roasted squash. Simmer for 20 minutes.
7 Using an immersion blender, puree until smooth.
8 Serve soup and garnish as desired.

NUTRITION INFORMATION
(per serving)
Calories: 183; Fat: 12g; Protein: 7g; Carbs: 12g; Fiber: 2g; Net Carbs: 10g

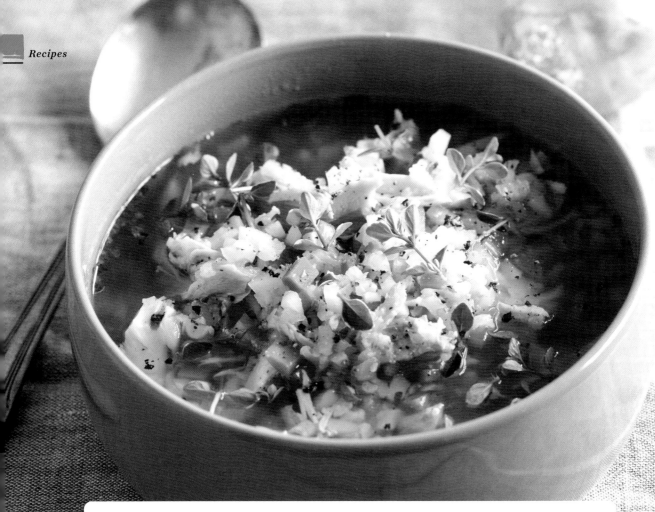

Chicken and Cauliflower Rice Soup

This comes together quickly so it's perfect for when things get hectic leading up to the holidays. It also makes a big batch, so you'll have leftovers for keto-friendly lunches.

PREP 15 minutes
TOTAL 35 minutes
SERVINGS 10

Ingredients

2 cups cooked, shredded chicken
6 cups chicken stock
2 cups chopped carrots
1 cup chopped celery
1 cup chopped onion
2 teaspoons minced garlic
2 bay leaves
1 tablespoon chopped parsley
¼ teaspoon dried thyme
½ teaspoon salt
½ teaspoon ground black pepper
2 cups riced cauliflower
Garnish: thyme sprigs

Instructions

1 In a Dutch oven, add all ingredients except the riced cauliflower.
2 Bring to a boil over medium-high heat. Reduce heat and simmer 5 minutes.
3 Add the riced cauliflower and cook another 5 minutes.
4 Remove and discard the bay leaves.
5 Serve soup and garnish as desired.

NUTRITION INFORMATION (per serving)
Calories: 355; Fat: 25g; Protein: 25g; Carbs: 5g; Fiber: 1g; Net Carbs: 4g

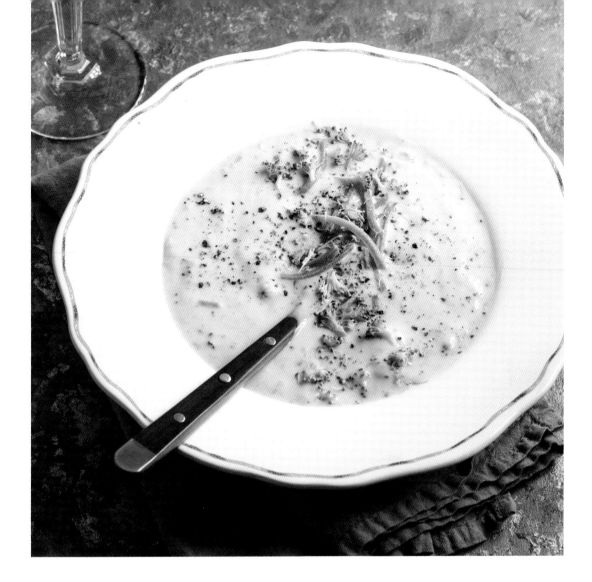

Broccoli Cheddar Soup

The classic combo is super-filling and an excellent substitute for the original carb-filled version!

PREP 10 minutes
TOTAL 20 minutes
SERVINGS 4

Ingredients

- 2   tablespoons butter
- ¼   cup chopped onion
- 1   teaspoon minced garlic
- 2   cups chicken stock
- ½   teaspoon salt
- ½   teaspoon ground black pepper
- 1   cup chopped broccoli
- 1   tablespoon cream cheese, softened
- ⅓   cup heavy cream
- 1   cup shredded Cheddar cheese
      Garnishes: chopped broccoli, shredded carrots, cracked black pepper

Instructions

1 In a Dutch oven, melt butter over medium-high heat. Sauté onion and garlic for 5 minutes.
2 Add the stock, salt, pepper and broccoli, and cook 1 minute. Add the cream cheese, cream and Cheddar cheese, and stir until melted.
3 Serve soup and garnish as desired.

NUTRITION INFORMATION (per serving)
Calories: 241; Fat: 18g; Protein: 10g; Carbs: 5g; Fiber: 1g; Net Carbs: 4g

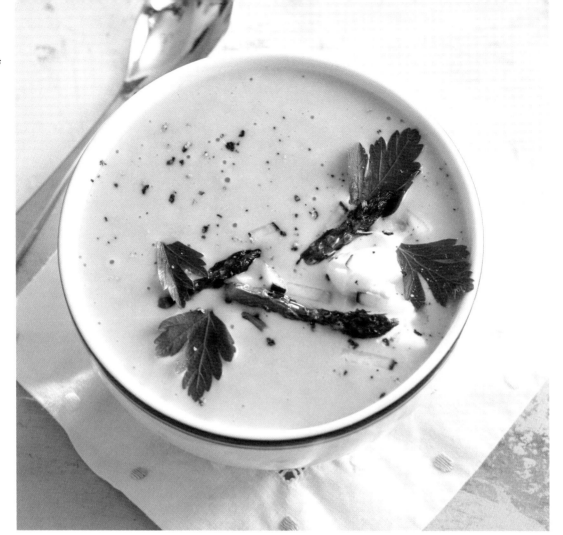

Cream of Asparagus Soup

For an elegant way to start off a holiday meal, look no further than this comforting soup. Top it with a dollop of Greek yogurt or sour cream for an even creamier texture.

PREP 15 minutes
TOTAL 30 minutes
SERVINGS 4

Ingredients

2 tablespoons butter
1 teaspoon minced garlic
2 tablespoons chopped onion
1½ cups asparagus pieces
3 cups vegetable broth
½ cup heavy cream
½ teaspoon sea salt
½ teaspoon ground black pepper
Garnishes: parsley leaves, asparagus pieces, sour cream, julienned radishes

Instructions

1 In a Dutch oven, heat the butter over low-medium heat. Add the garlic and onion and cook for 3 minutes.
2 Stir in the asparagus pieces and cook for 5 minutes.
3 Add the vegetable broth and bring to a boil. Reduce to a simmer for 5 minutes.
4 Using an immersion blender, blend until smooth. Stir in the cream, salt and pepper.
5 Serve soup and garnish as desired.

NUTRITION INFORMATION (per serving)
Calories: 155; Fat: 14g; Protein: 3g; Carbs: 5g; Fiber: 1g; Net Carbs: 4g

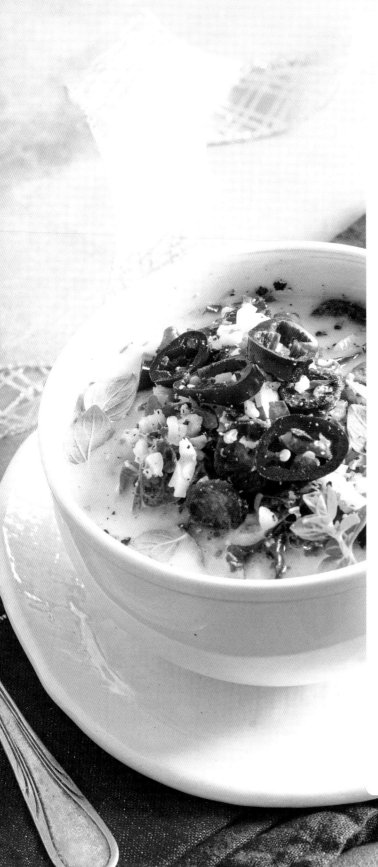

Turkey Sausage and Kale Soup

In this take on the classic Zuppa Toscana, cauliflower is substituted for potatoes to keep this version low-carb!

PREP 10 minutes
TOTAL 20 minutes
SERVINGS 8

Ingredients

- 1 pound turkey kielbasa sausage, sliced
- ½ cup chopped onion
- 2 tablespoons minced garlic
- 8 cups chicken broth
- ¼ cup lemon juice
- 1 tablespoon dried oregano
- 3 cups riced cauliflower
- ½ cup heavy cream
- 1 bunch kale, chopped
- ½ teaspoon sea salt
- ½ teaspoon ground black pepper
  Garnishes: oregano leaves, sliced Fresno peppers

Instructions

1 In a Dutch oven, sauté the sausage and onion for 5 minutes. Stir in the garlic and cook 1 more minute.
2 Add the chicken broth, lemon juice, oregano and riced cauliflower. Bring to a low boil.
3 Reduce the heat and simmer for 10 minutes or until the cauliflower is tender.
4 Stir in the heavy cream, kale, salt and pepper and let sit for 5 minutes until kale is wilted.
5 Serve soup and garnish as desired.

NUTRITION INFORMATION
(per serving)
Calories: 275; Fat: 18g; Protein: 15g; Carbs: 8g; Fiber: 2g; Net Carbs: 6g

Entrées

Time for the main course! Dish up elegant yet easy mains that are sure to impress.

Whole Roasted Chicken With Radishes

The scent of roasting chicken will bring everyone to the dinner table.

PREP 10 minutes
TOTAL 1 hour 10 minutes +
10 minutes inactive
SERVINGS 6

Ingredients

- 1 (5-pound) whole chicken
- 1 tablespoon olive oil
- 1 tablespoon salt
- 1 teaspoon ground black pepper
- 1 teaspoon minced garlic
- 1 large onion, quartered
- 1 bunch radishes, halved
  Garnish: sage leaves

Instructions

1 Preheat oven to 375°F.
2 Brush chicken with olive oil; sprinkle with salt, pepper and garlic.
3 Place chicken in roasting pan and truss legs with kitchen twine. Arrange the vegetables around chicken.
4 Roast for 50 to 60 minutes or until meat thermometer registers an internal temperature of 165°F.
5 Remove from oven; let chicken rest for 10 minutes.
6 Transfer to serving platter; garnish as desired.

NUTRITION INFORMATION (per serving)
Calories: 330; Fat: 18g; Protein: 32g;
Carbs: 5g; Fiber: 2g; Net Carbs: 3g

Pork Chops With Pesto

On days when your holiday prep is cutting into your dinner prep, skillet-cooked pork chops make for a delicious, simple option.

PREP 5 minutes
TOTAL 15 minutes
SERVINGS 2

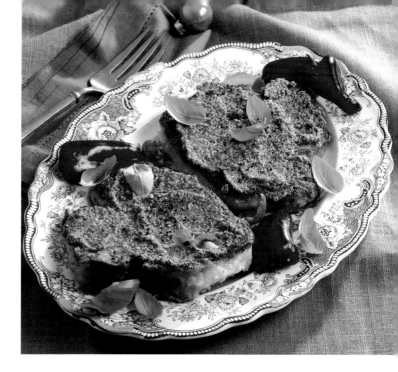

Ingredients

- 2 tablespoons almond flour
- 1 teaspoon sea salt
- ½ teaspoon ground black pepper
- 2 8-ounce boneless pork chops
  Vegetable oil cooking spray
- 2 tablespoons pesto
  Garnishes: halved baby red bell peppers, basil leaves

Instructions

1 In a shallow dish, combine almond flour, salt and pepper.
2 Dredge both sides of each pork chop in the flour mixture.
3 Coat a large skillet with vegetable oil cooking spray; preheat over medium-high heat.
4 Brown the pork chops for 2 minutes on each side.
5 Spread pesto on one side of each chop; cover skillet and continue cooking for an additional 2 minutes or until meat thermometer registers an internal temperature of 160°F.
6 Transfer to serving platter; garnish as desired.

NUTRITION INFORMATION (per serving)
Calories: 350; Fat: 16g; Protein: 36g;
Carbs: 10g; Fiber: 3g; Net Carbs: 7g

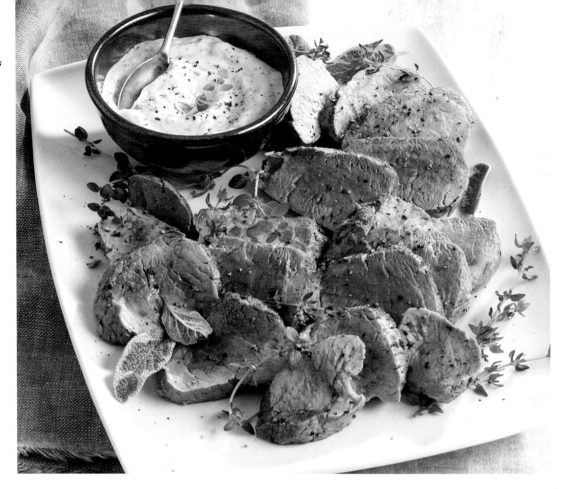

Pork Tenderloin With Mustard Sauce

Try this savory dish for a special holiday dinner or serve it on New Year's Day.

PREP 10 minutes
TOTAL 35 minutes + 40 minutes inactive
SERVINGS 6

Ingredients

1½ pounds pork tenderloin
1 tablespoon olive oil
2 tablespoons Dijon mustard
1 teaspoon sea salt, divided
¾ teaspoon ground black pepper, divided
½ cup sour cream
2 tablespoons heavy cream
2 tablespoons stone-ground mustard
1 tablespoon prepared horseradish
1 tablespoon vegetable oil
Garnishes: thyme sprigs, sage leaves, oregano sprigs

Instructions

1 Place pork in a plastic zip-close bag. Add olive oil, Dijon mustard, ½ teaspoon salt and ¼ teaspoon pepper to bag. Seal bag; marinate pork for 30 minutes.

2 Meanwhile to make sauce, in a medium bowl, combine sour cream, heavy cream, stone-ground mustard, horseradish, and remaining salt and pepper.

3 In a cast-iron skillet over medium-high heat, heat the vegetable oil. Sear pork on all sides.

4 Place skillet in oven; roast pork for an additional 10 minutes or until pork reaches the desired degree of doneness.

5 Let pork rest on cutting board for 10 minutes, then slice.

6 Transfer to serving platter; garnish as desired and serve sauce on the side.

NUTRITION INFORMATION (per serving)
Calories: 335; Fat: 26g; Protein: 26g; Carbs: 2g; Fiber: 0g; Net Carbs: 2g

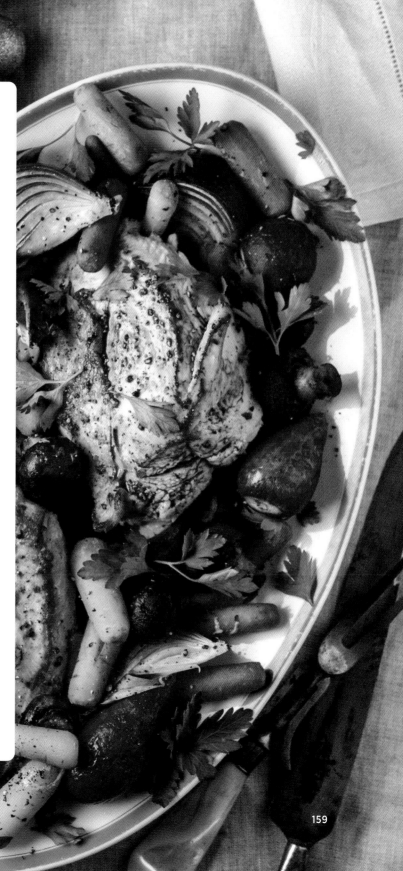

Roasted Turkey Breast With Vegetables

This simple preparation will make your holiday dinner party stress-free. If you'd like to serve gravy along with it, there are a number of keto-compliant gravy packets on the market.

PREP 10 minutes
TOTAL 2 hours + 20 minutes inactive
SERVINGS 8

Ingredients

- 2 (3 pounds each) bone-in turkey breast halves
- 2 tablespoons olive oil
- 1 cup baby carrots
- 1 cup radishes
- 1 cup baby portobello mushrooms
- 1 red onion, quartered
- ½ teaspoon sea salt
- ½ teaspoon ground black pepper
- Garnish: parsley leaves

Instructions

1 Preheat oven to 425°F.
2 Place turkey breasts in a roasting pan; brush with olive oil.
3 Arrange vegetables around turkey breasts; sprinkle with salt and pepper.
4 Reduce oven temperature to 375°F. Roast for 1½ hours or until meat thermometer registers an internal temperature of 165°F.
5 Remove from oven, cover with foil and let turkey stand 20 minutes before slicing.
6 Transfer to serving platter; garnish as desired.

NUTRITION INFORMATION
(per serving)
Calories: 310; Fat: 9g; Protein: 25g; Carbs: 6g; Fiber: 2g; Net Carbs: 4g

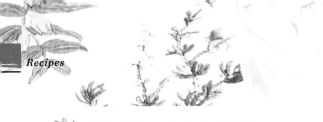

Beef Tenderloin With Horseradish Cream

This showstopping dish will impress your guests, and no one will even suspect it's "diet." Serve with keto-friendly veggies, like mashed cauliflower or creamed spinach.

PREP 15 minutes
TOTAL 1 hour
SERVINGS 8

Ingredients

- ½ cup sour cream
- 2 tablespoons prepared horseradish
- 3½ teaspoons sea salt, divided
- 2½ teaspoons cracked black pepper, divided
- 1 teaspoon minced garlic
- 1 (3-pound) center-cut beef tenderloin
- 1 tablespoon olive oil
- 1 tablespoon butter
- 1 head garlic, halved
- 2 shallots, halved
- 1 bunch thyme
  Garnishes: thyme sprigs, grape tomatoes

Instructions

1 In a medium bowl, whisk together sour cream, horseradish, ½ teaspoon salt and ½ teaspoon pepper until smooth. Cover and refrigerate for up to 2 days.
2 Preheat oven to 400°F.
3 In a small bowl, combine garlic and remaining salt and pepper. Rub mixture all over tenderloin.
4 In a large skillet, heat the olive oil and butter over medium-high heat. Brown the meat on all sides, about 5 minutes. Add garlic and shallots to skillet; cook for 2 minutes.
5 Place thyme bunch in the bottom of a large roasting pan. Add the meat, garlic and shallots to pan.
6 Roast for 30 minutes. Transfer to cutting board. Let rest for 15 minutes before slicing.
7 Transfer to serving platter; garnish as desired and serve horseradish cream on the side.

NUTRITION INFORMATION (per serving)
Calories: 550; Fat: 40g; Protein: 38g; Carbs: 8g; Fiber: 2g; Net Carbs: 6g

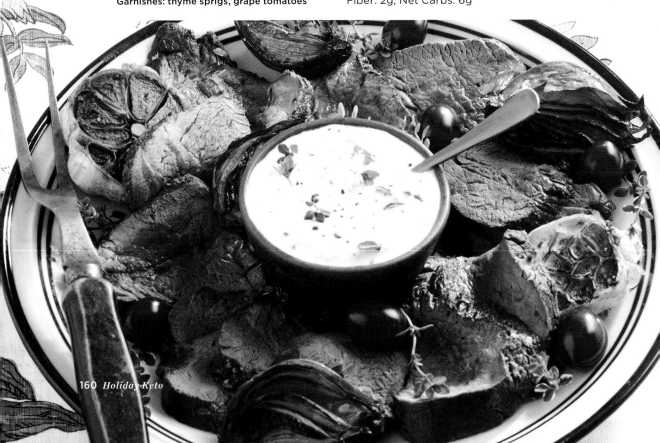

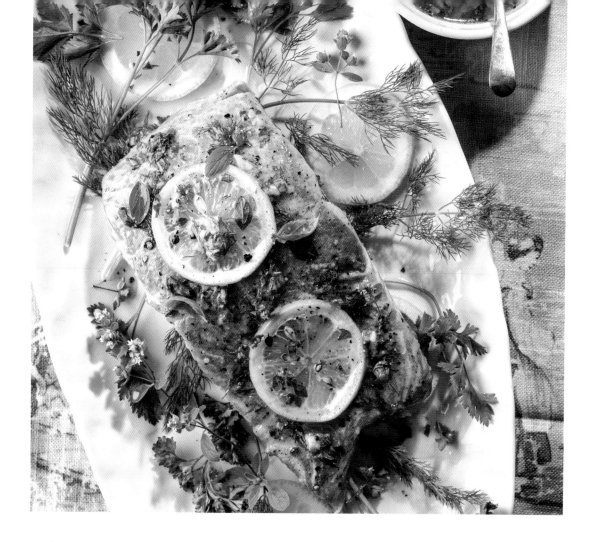

Baked Salmon With Lemon and Herbs

Salmon is one of the healthiest fish, making this dish ideal for holiday dinner parties or to serve year-round.

PREP 5 minutes

TOTAL 20 minutes

SERVINGS 4

Ingredients

- ¼ cup butter, divided
- 1 teaspoon minced garlic
- 2 tablespoons chopped parsley
- ½ teaspoon sea salt
- ¼ teaspoon ground black pepper
- 2 pounds salmon fillets, cut into 4 portions
- 1 large lemon, sliced

Garnishes: lemon slices, basil leaves, parsley sprigs, thyme sprigs, oregano sprigs

Instructions

1 Preheat oven to 400°F.

2 Place 2 tablespoons butter on a rimmed baking sheet. Place in oven to melt.

3 In a small bowl, melt the remaining butter; whisk in garlic, parsley, salt and pepper.

4 Remove baking pan from oven; place salmon fillets, skin-side down, on pan. Arrange lemon slices on fillets and pour garlic butter over top.

5 Roast for 10 to 12 minutes, until the fish is cooked to desired doneness.

6 Transfer to serving platter; spoon garlic butter from pan onto fillets and garnish as desired.

NUTRITION INFORMATION (per serving)
Calories: 266; Fat: 13g; Protein: 34g; Carbs: 2g; Fiber: 1g; Net Carbs: 1g

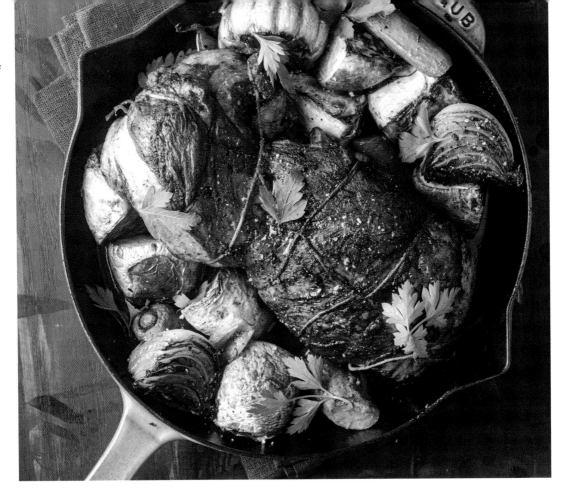

Leg of Lamb With Root Vegetables

Let this roasted dish be the centerpiece of your table for a holiday dinner party.

PREP 15 minutes
TOTAL 1 hour 15 minutes + 15 minutes inactive
SERVINGS 8

Ingredients

- 1 (6-pound) boneless leg of lamb, tied
- 4 teaspoons sea salt, divided
- 1 teaspoon ground black pepper
- ½ cup Dijon mustard
- ¼ cup Italian seasoning
- 2 large red onions, quartered
- 4 carrots, peeled and cut into large chunks
- 2 turnips, quartered
- 1 head garlic, halved
- 2 tablespoons olive oil
- 1 cup beef stock
  Garnish: parsley leaves

Instructions

1 Preheat oven to 400°F.
2 Sprinkle lamb with 1 tablespoon sea salt and pepper. Coat lamb with Dijon mustard and Italian seasoning. Place lamb in roasting pan.
3 Arrange vegetables in pan around lamb. Drizzle with olive oil; sprinkle with remaining 1 teaspoon salt.
4 Pour in beef stock. Cover pan with foil.
5 Roast for 45 minutes to 1 hour. Remove foil and increase temperature to 425°F.
6 Roast an additional 15 minutes or until meat thermometer registers an internal temperature of 130°F.
7 Remove from oven; let lamb rest for 15 minutes before slicing.
8 Transfer to serving platter; garnish as desired.

NUTRITION INFORMATION (per serving)
Calories: 450; Fat: 14g; Protein: 45g; Carbs: 8g; Fiber: 4g; Net Carbs: 4g

Slow-Cooker Beef Brisket

Slow cooking turns a cut of meat that can be tough into a fork-tender meal. It can be made ahead, so it's ideal for parties and potlucks.

PREP 20 minutes
TOTAL 4 hours 20 minutes
SERVINGS 8

Ingredients

- 1 tablespoon garlic powder
- 1 tablespoon onion powder
- 2 teaspoons paprika
- 1 teaspoon salt
- 1 teaspoon ground black pepper
- 4 pounds beef brisket, at room temperature
- 2 tablespoons olive oil
- 2 cups beef stock
- ½ cup dry red wine

Garnishes: rosemary sprigs, tomato slices

Instructions

1 In a small bowl, combine the garlic powder, onion powder, paprika, salt and pepper. Rub the mixture all over the brisket.

2 In a large skillet, heat the olive oil over medium-high heat; brown meat on both sides.

3 Place the meat in slow cooker; pour stock and wine over meat.

4 Cook on High for 4 hours or until tender.

5 Slice meat and transfer to serving platter; garnish as desired.

NUTRITION INFORMATION (per serving)
Calories: 244; Fat: 12g; Protein: 32g; Carbs: 1g; Fiber: 0g; Net Carbs: 1g

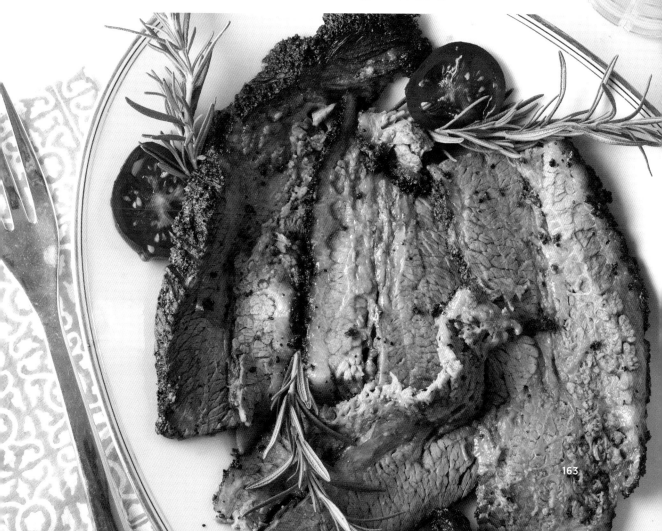

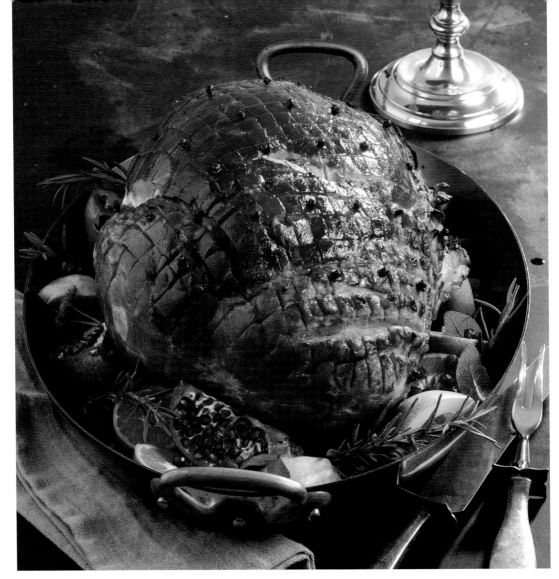

Bourbon Baked Ham

A glazed ham is a holiday classic, and the bourbon in this glaze imparts a rich flavor.

PREP 10 minutes
TOTAL 2 hours 10 minutes
SERVINGS 12

Ingredients

- 1 (18-pound) fully cooked, semi-boneless ham
- 1 tablespoon whole cloves
- ½ cup butter
- ½ cup bourbon
- ⅓ cup Truvia brown sugar substitute
  Garnishes: sage sprigs, rosemary sprigs, tangerines, pomegranates, pears

Instructions

1 Preheat oven to 350°F.
2 Use a sharp knife to score the ham in a crisscross pattern. Stick whole cloves into ham where scored lines cross.
3 Grease a large roasting pan; place ham in pan.
4 In a small saucepan, heat the butter, bourbon and brown sugar substitute; stir until smooth.
5 Pour mixture over ham.
6 Bake ham for 2 hours, basting frequently.
7 Transfer to serving platter; garnish as desired.

NUTRITION INFORMATION (per serving)
Calories: 434; Fat: 24g; Protein: 45g; Carbs: 0g; Fiber: 0g; Net Carbs: 0g

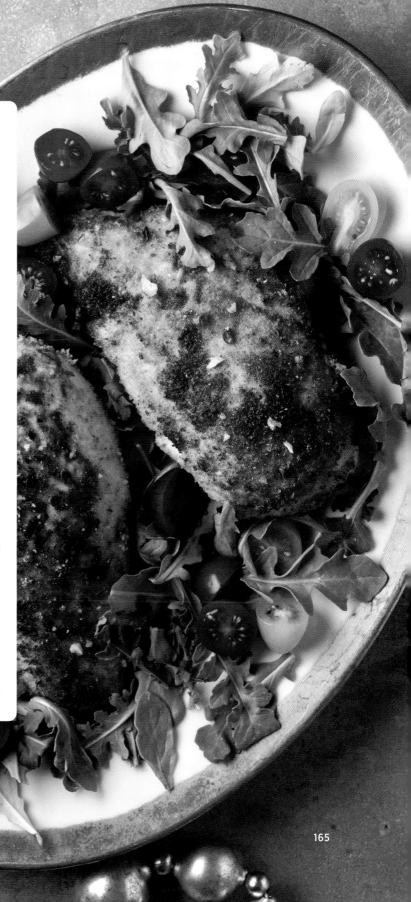

Pistachio-Crusted Chicken Breasts

Pistachios provide a tasty crunch and healthy fats to this meal.

PREP 10 minutes
TOTAL 45 minutes
SERVINGS 2

Ingredients

- ½ cup pistachios
- ½ cup almond flour
- 2 boneless, skinless chicken breasts, about 1½ inches thick
- 2 tablespoons mustard
  Vegetable oil cooking spray
  Garnishes: arugula, cherry tomatoes

Instructions

1 Preheat oven to 400°F.
2 In a food processor, pulse the pistachios until they have the texture of breadcrumbs.
3 In a shallow dish, combine the pistachios and almond flour.
4 Brush both sides of each chicken breast with mustard. Dip chicken into pistachio mixture, pressing to adhere.
5 Coat baking sheet with vegetable oil cooking spray. Place chicken on sheet.
6 Bake 25 to 35 minutes or until cooked through.
7 Transfer to serving platter; garnish as desired.

NUTRITION INFORMATION

(per serving)
Calories: 441; Fat: 23g; Protein: 49g; Carbs: 7g; Fiber: 3g; Net Carbs: 4g

Sides

Make your mark!
These crowd-pleasing side dishes are surprisingly low-carb.

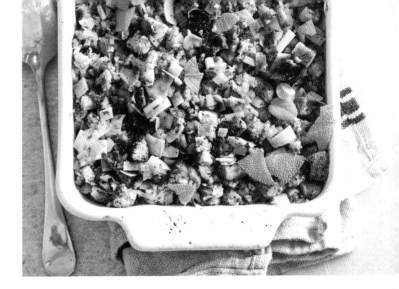

Creamy Mushrooms With Thyme

Use your favorite mushrooms, or try a mixture, for a delicious side dish.

PREP 5 minutes
TOTAL 25 minutes
SERVINGS 4

Ingredients

- 2   slices bacon
- 1   teaspoon minced garlic
- 1   tablespoon chopped onion
- 1½ cups assorted mushrooms, sliced
- 2   tablespoons cream cheese
- 1   tablespoon grated Parmesan cheese
- 1   teaspoon Dijon mustard
- 1   tablespoon heavy cream
- ¼   cup vegetable broth
     Garnishes: thyme sprigs, cracked black pepper

Instructions

1 In a large skillet, cook the bacon over medium-high until crisp, about 8 minutes.
2 Remove bacon (leave the fat) from the skillet and chop.
3 Add garlic and onion to skillet; cook for 2 minutes.
4 Add mushrooms to skillet; cook for 3 more minutes.
5 Add cream cheese, Parmesan cheese, mustard, cream and broth; cook until thickened.
6 Pour into serving bowl; top with reserved bacon. Garnish as desired.

NUTRITION INFORMATION (per serving)
Calories: 325; Fat: 27g; Protein: 6g; Carbs: 3g; Fiber: 1g; Net Carbs: 2g

---

Savory Sage Stuffing

This will be a huge hit at your holiday table! Double it if you're serving a crowd.

PREP 10 minutes
TOTAL 30 minutes
SERVINGS 4

Ingredients

- 4   slices keto bread, crumbled
- 3   tablespoons olive oil, divided
- 2   stalks celery, chopped
- 1   leek, chopped
- 1   teaspoon minced garlic
- 1   teaspoon chopped parsley
- 1   teaspoon chopped sage
- ¼   cup melted butter
- ½   teaspoon sea salt
- ¼   teaspoon ground black pepper
- ½   cup chicken broth
     Garnish: torn sage leaves

Instructions

1 Preheat oven to 350°F.
2 On a baking sheet, spread the bread crumbles. Drizzle with 2 tablespoons olive oil.
3 Bake for 5 minutes or until lightly browned.
4 In a large skillet over medium-high heat, add remaining 1 tablespoon olive oil. Stir in celery, leek, garlic, parsley and sage; sauté for 2 minutes. Remove from heat.
5 Stir in melted butter, salt, pepper and broth. Add bread crumbles; stir just to combine.
6 Place mixture in an 8-inch baking dish; bake, covered, for 15 minutes.
7 Garnish as desired before serving.

NUTRITION INFORMATION (per serving)
Calories: 127; Fat: 9g; Protein: 4g; Carbs: 8g; Fiber: 2g; Net Carbs: 6g

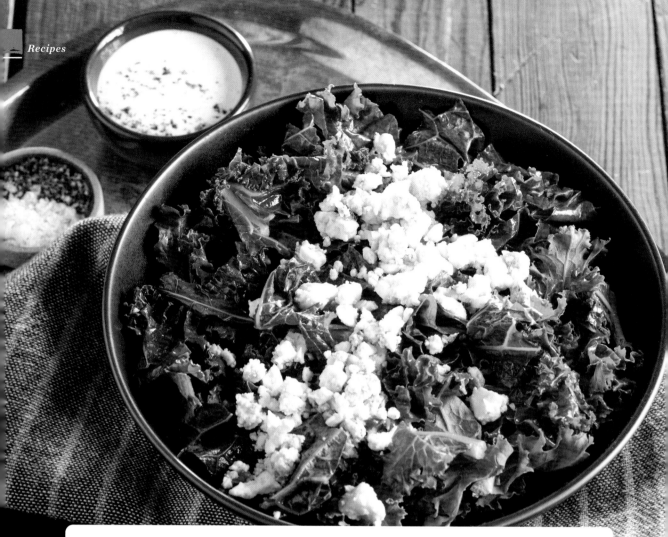

Warm Kale With Gorgonzola

This warm, tangy accompaniment is perfect with a simple grilled steak. (Top the steak with additional gorgonzola, too!)

PREP 10 minutes
TOTAL 15 minutes
SERVINGS 4

Ingredients

- ¾ cup heavy cream
- 3 tablespoons mayonnaise
- 1 tablespoon Dijon mustard
- 2 tablespoons olive oil
- 1 teaspoon minced garlic
- 2 tablespoons butter
- 8 ounces kale, trimmed
- ½ teaspoon salt
- ½ teaspoon ground black pepper
- ¼ cup crumbled gorgonzola cheese

Instructions

1 In a small bowl to make dressing, mix together cream, mayonnaise, mustard, olive oil and garlic.
2 In a large skillet over medium-high heat, melt butter. Add kale to skillet; sauté for 1 to 2 minutes. Sprinkle with salt and pepper.
3 Place kale in serving bowl, and pour dressing over kale.
4 Sprinkle with crumbled gorgonzola cheese before serving.

NUTRITION INFORMATION (per serving)
Calories: 450; Fat: 38g; Protein: 8g; Carbs: 7g; Fiber: 2g; Net Carbs: 5g

Whipped Cauliflower Mash

You'll love this side with any of your main courses. If you're serving it to company, you may want to make a double batch; it's so delicious that even non-ketoers won't be able to resist a heaping serving!

PREP 5 minutes
TOTAL 15 minutes
SERVINGS 4

Ingredients

- 6 cups water
- 1 large head cauliflower, cut into florets
- 1 tablespoon minced garlic
- ¼ cup grated Parmesan cheese
- 2 tablespoons butter
- ½ teaspoon sea salt
- ½ teaspoon ground black pepper

Garnishes: chopped chives, cracked black pepper

Instructions

1 Add water to large pot and boil, then add cauliflower. Boil until tender, 8 to 10 minutes.
2 Reserve 1 cup of cooking liquid, then drain cauliflower.
3 In a blender, combine cauliflower, garlic, Parmesan cheese, butter, salt and pepper; blend until smooth. (If the mash is too thick, slowly add reserved cooking liquid to obtain the desired consistency.)
4 Pour cauliflower mash into serving bowl, and garnish as desired.

NUTRITION INFORMATION (per serving)
Calories: 128; Fat: 8g; Protein: 4g; Carbs: 11g; Fiber: 4g; Net Carbs: 7g

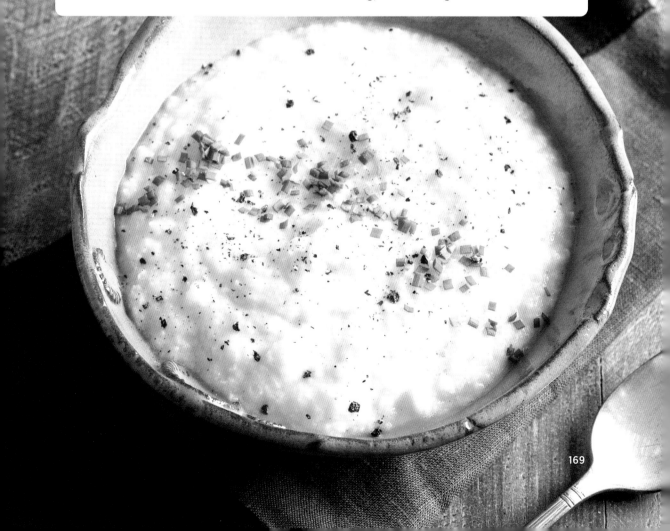

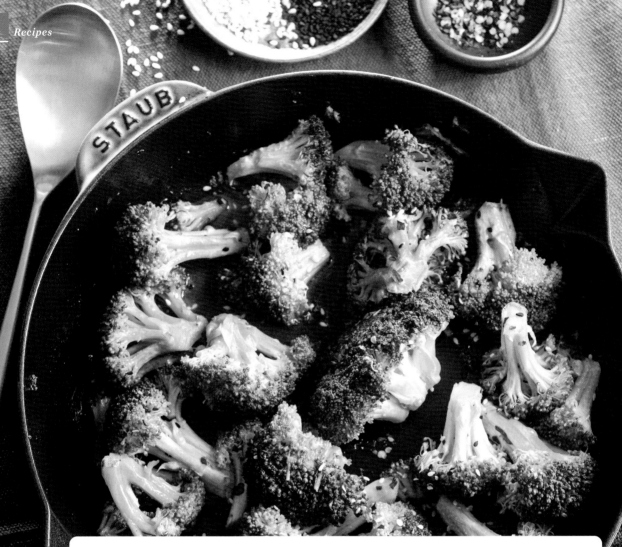

Sesame Broccoli

This quick and easy side dish pairs well with Asian-inspired beef. You can substitute asparagus or snow peas for the broccoli, or add some chile oil to spice things up.

PREP 5 minutes
TOTAL 15 minutes
SERVINGS 4

Ingredients

2   tablespoons sesame oil
1   teaspoon minced garlic
1   (12-ounce) bag broccoli florets
2   tablespoons water
1   tablespoon toasted sesame seeds
½   teaspoon red pepper flakes
¼   cup light gluten-free soy sauce

Instructions

1 In a large skillet over medium-high heat, heat sesame oil. Stir in garlic; cook for 1 minute.
2 Add broccoli to the skillet; cook for 1 minute.
3 Reduce heat to medium; add water. Cook for 3 to 4 minutes or until water has evaporated.
4 Sprinkle with sesame seeds and red pepper flakes; cook for 1 minute.
5 Stir in soy sauce before serving.

NUTRITION INFORMATION (per serving)
Calories: 120; Fat: 7g; Protein: 4g; Carbs: 9g; Fiber: 3g; Net Carbs: 6g

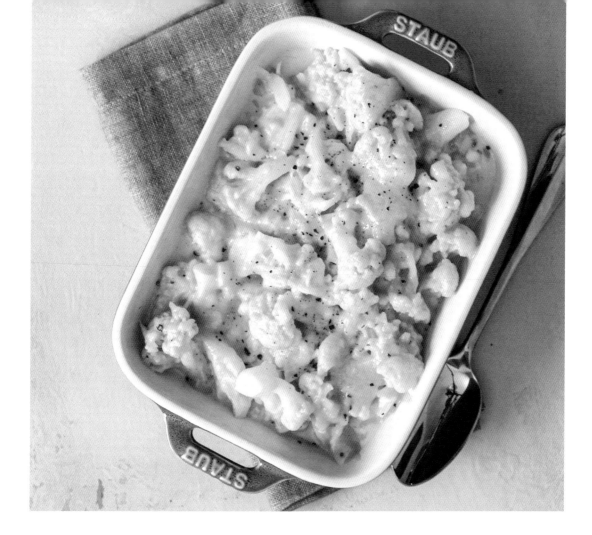

"Mac" and Cheese

This one is so creamy and satisfying you'll find
yourself preparing it for a light lunch as well as
for a dinner side.

PREP 5 minutes
TOTAL 25 minutes
SERVINGS 4

Ingredients

      Vegetable oil cooking spray
  4   cups cauliflower florets
  ¼   cup melted butter
  ½   teaspoon salt
  ½   teaspoon ground black pepper
  1   cup shredded Cheddar cheese
  ⅓   cup heavy cream
  ¼   cup milk

Garnishes: shredded Cheddar cheese, cracked
black pepper

Instructions

1 Preheat oven to 450°F. Spray a baking sheet
with vegetable oil cooking spray.
2 In a large bowl, toss cauliflower florets, melted
butter, salt and pepper.
3 Place cauliflower on baking sheet; roast for
15 minutes or until tender.
4 In a glass bowl, combine Cheddar cheese,
cream and milk. Microwave mixture until melted,
about 1 minute.
5 Toss cauliflower with cheese mixture, place into
casserole dish and bake at 350°F for 5 minutes.
6 Garnish as desired to serve.

NUTRITION INFORMATION (per serving)
Calories: 294; Fat: 23g; Protein: 11g; Carbs: 12g;
Fiber: 5g; Net Carbs: 7g

Cranberry Sauce

This sugar-free version of the holiday classic is just as delicious as the original.

PREP 5 minutes
TOTAL 20 minutes
SERVINGS 6

Ingredients

- 1 (12-ounce) bag cranberries
- 1 cup powdered erythritol
- ¾ cup water
- 1 tablespoon orange juice
- 1 teaspoon orange zest
- ½ teaspoon vanilla extract
  Garnish: orange zest

Instructions

1 In a medium saucepan, combine cranberries, erythritol, water, orange juice and orange zest.
2 Bring to a boil, then reduce heat to a simmer.
3 Simmer for 12 to 15 minutes, or until berries burst and sauce thickens.
4 Remove from heat; stir in vanilla extract.
5 Cool and serve immediately, or refrigerate until serving.
6 Pour cranberry sauce into a bowl, and garnish as desired to serve.

NUTRITION INFORMATION (per serving)
Calories: 44; Fat: 0g; Protein: 0g; Carbs: 8g; Fiber: 4g; Net Carbs: 4g

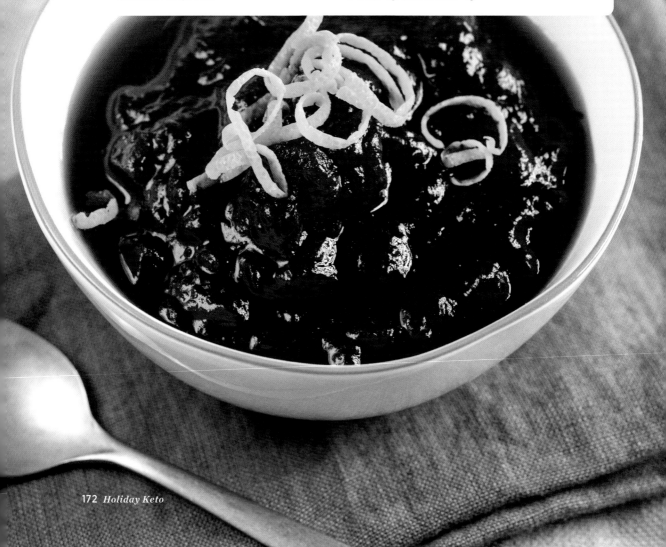

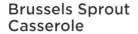

Brussels Sprout Casserole

These creamy, nutty sprouts will be the highlight of your holiday meal.

PREP 10 minutes
TOTAL 20 minutes
SERVINGS 6

Ingredients

- 2 tablespoons butter
- 1 cup chopped onion
- 1 tablespoon minced garlic
- 1 pound fresh Brussels sprouts, trimmed and halved
- 1 teaspoon sea salt
- ½ teaspoon ground black pepper
- 2 tablespoons cream cheese
- ⅓ cup heavy cream
- ½ cup toasted pecans, chopped

Instructions

1 In a large skillet over medium-high heat, melt butter.
2 Add onion and garlic; cook for 3 minutes.
3 Stir in Brussels sprouts, salt and pepper; cook for 3 minutes.
4 Stir in cream cheese and heavy cream; cook for 2 minutes or until thickened.
5 Place in serving dish; top with chopped pecans.

NUTRITION INFORMATION
(per serving)
Calories: 225; Fat: 6g; Protein: 5g; Carbs: 7g; Fiber: 3g; Net Carbs: 4g

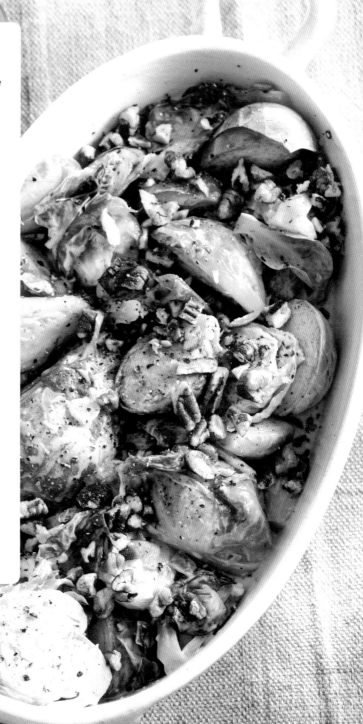

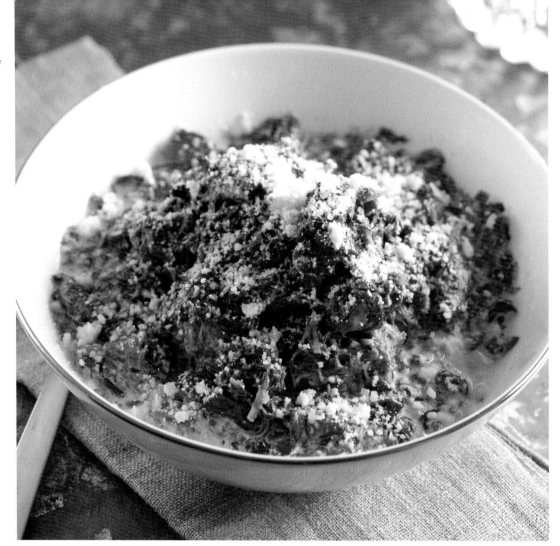

Creamed Spinach With Nutmeg

A pinch of nutmeg enhances the creaminess of this dish—a steakhouse classic that's bound to become a new holiday staple.

PREP 5 minutes
TOTAL 15 minutes
SERVINGS 4

Ingredients

¼ cup butter

1 tablespoon minced garlic

1 (10-ounce) bag spinach (about 16 cups)

½ cup heavy cream

4 ounces cream cheese, softened

½ teaspoon sea salt

¼ teaspoon ground black pepper

⅛ teaspoon grated nutmeg

Garnish: grated Parmesan cheese

Instructions

1 In a large skillet over medium-high heat, melt the butter.

2 Add garlic to skillet; sauté for 1 minute.

3 Add spinach to skillet; sauté for 3 minutes or until wilted.

4 Add heavy cream, cream cheese, salt, pepper and nutmeg.

5 Stir until smooth and heated through.

6 Pour spinach into bowl, and garnish as desired.

NUTRITION INFORMATION (per serving)
Calories: 274; Fat: 25g; Protein: 4g; Carbs: 5g; Fiber: 1g; Net Carbs: 4g

Sautéed Cabbage with Bacon

Try serving this alongside some grilled pork chops for a hearty, keto-friendly meal that's sure to please bacon lovers!

PREP 5 minutes
TOTAL 20 minutes
SERVINGS 4

Ingredients

- ¼ cup butter
- 1 teaspoon minced garlic
- 1½ pounds cabbage, shredded
- ½ teaspoon sea salt
- ½ teaspoon ground black pepper
- Garnish: crumbled bacon

Instructions

1 In a large skillet over medium-high heat, melt the butter.
2 Stir in the garlic and cook for 30 seconds. Add the cabbage; sauté for 15 minutes, stirring occasionally, until the cabbage is wilted.
3 Sprinkle with salt and pepper. Pour cabbage into bowl, and garnish as desired.

NUTRITION INFORMATION (per serving)
Calories: 153; Fat: 4.5g; Protein: 3g; Carbs: 10.5g; Fiber: 4g; Net Carbs: 6.5g

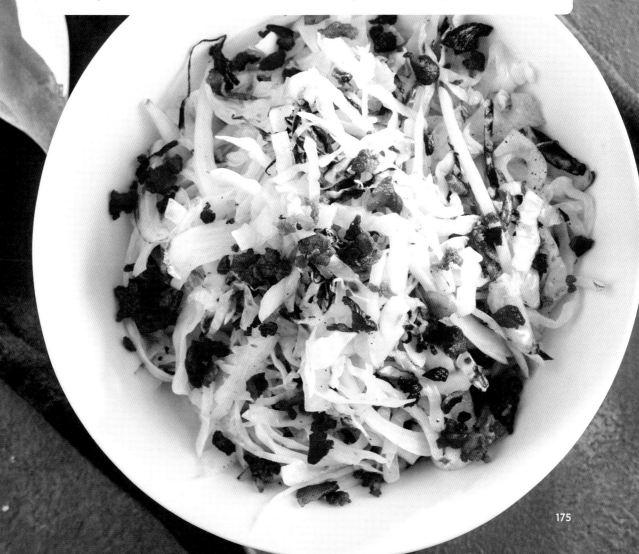

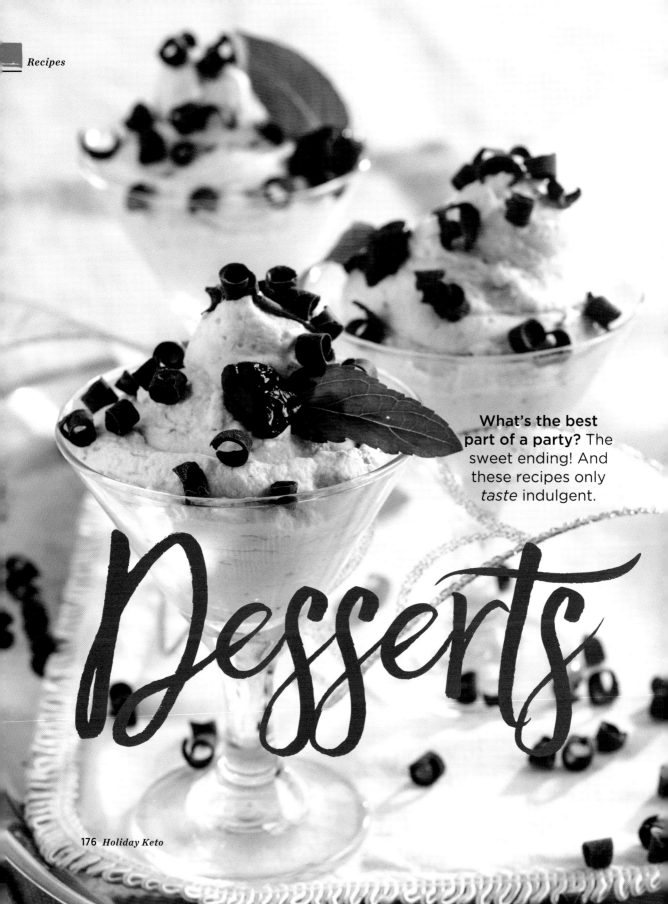

What's the best part of a party? The sweet ending! And these recipes only *taste* indulgent.

Desserts

Cranberry Mousse

If you make this dessert before you start dinner, it'll be chilled and ready by the time you're done with the main course.

PREP 5 minutes
TOTAL 5 minutes + 20 minutes inactive
SERVINGS 4

Ingredients

1½   cups heavy whipping cream
⅓   cup smooth cranberry sauce
4   ounces cream cheese, softened
      Garnishes: dried cranberries, mint leaves, shaved unsweetened dark chocolate

Instructions

1 In a mixing bowl, use a hand mixer to beat heavy cream for 2 minutes or until stiff peaks form.
2 In another bowl, beat cranberry sauce and cream cheese together until smooth.
3 Fold cranberry mixture into whipped cream until just combined.
4 Spoon mousse into individual serving bowls; refrigerate for at least 20 minutes.
5 Garnish as desired to serve.

NUTRITION INFORMATION (per serving)
Calories: 215; Fat: 20g; Protein: 4g; Carbs: 6g; Fiber: 2g; Net Carbs: 4g

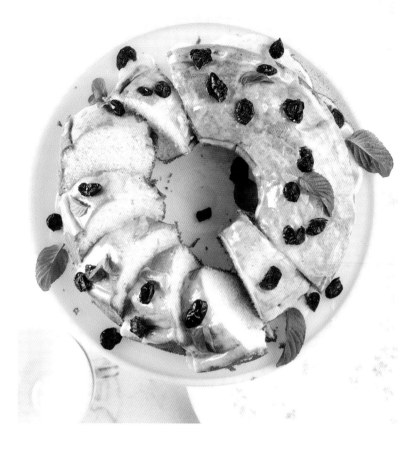

Spiced Vanilla Cake

This spiced cake is the perfect finish to a decadent meal.

PREP 15 minutes
TOTAL 45 minutes
SERVINGS 10

Ingredients

4   ounces cream cheese, softened
½   cup butter, softened
½   cup granulated sugar substitute (stevia)
¼   teaspoon allspice
⅛   teaspoon salt
½   teaspoon baking powder
5   eggs, beaten
1   teaspoon vanilla
2   cups almond flour
½   cup powdered sugar substitute (stevia)
2   tablespoons heavy cream
      Garnishes: dried cranberries, mint leaves

Instructions

1 Preheat oven to 350°F. Grease a small tube pan.
2 In a large mixing bowl, use a hand mixer to beat cream cheese and butter until smooth.
3 Add stevia, allspice, salt, baking powder, eggs, vanilla and almond flour; beat well.
4 Pour batter into prepared pan. Bake for 20 to 30 minutes, or until knife inserted in center comes out clean and edges begin to brown.
5 In a small bowl, whisk together the powdered stevia and heavy cream until smooth.
6 Drizzle glaze over cake; garnish as desired.

NUTRITION INFORMATION (per serving)
Calories: 224; Fat: 21g; Protein: 5g; Carbs: 18g; Fiber: 1g; Net Carbs: 17g

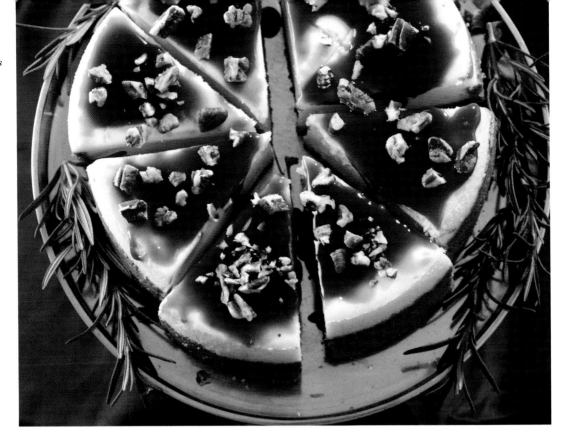

Butter Pecan Cheesecake

This rich, creamy dessert is sure to wow everyone at your holiday table.

PREP 30 minutes
TOTAL 1 hour 20 minutes + 2 hours inactive
SERVINGS 10

Ingredients

- 2 cups pecans
- 6 tablespoons butter
- 2 teaspoons vanilla extract
- ¼ cup monk fruit sweetener
- 2 (8-ounce) packages cream cheese, softened
- 1¼ cups heavy cream
- ¼ cup stevia
- ¼ cup low-sugar caramel sauce
- ¼ cup chopped pecans
- ½ teaspoon sea salt
  Garnish: rosemary sprigs

Instructions

1 Preheat oven to 350°F.
2 In a food processor, process the pecans until finely ground.
3 In a large bowl, combine ground pecans, butter, 1 teaspoon vanilla extract and monk fruit sweetener.
4 Line the bottom of an 8-inch springform pan with a parchment round.
5 Spoon pecan mixture into the prepared pan, pressing down to form an even crust. Refrigerate until ready to fill.
6 In a large mixing bowl, use a hand mixer to beat cream cheese until smooth.
7 Beat in cream, stevia and remaining 1 teaspoon vanilla extract until smooth.
8 Pour mixture evenly into prepared pan; bake for 45 to 50 minutes or until center is almost set, but still jiggly.
9 Let cheesecake cool to room temperature, about 2 hours.
10 Run a knife around the edge of cheesecake to remove it from pan. Place on serving dish.
11 Chill cheesecake until ready to serve. Top with caramel sauce and sprinkle with chopped pecans and sea salt; garnish with rosemary, if desired.

NUTRITION INFORMATION (per serving)
Calories: 303; Fat: 28g; Protein: 7g; Carbs: 4g; Fiber: 1g; Net Carbs: 3g

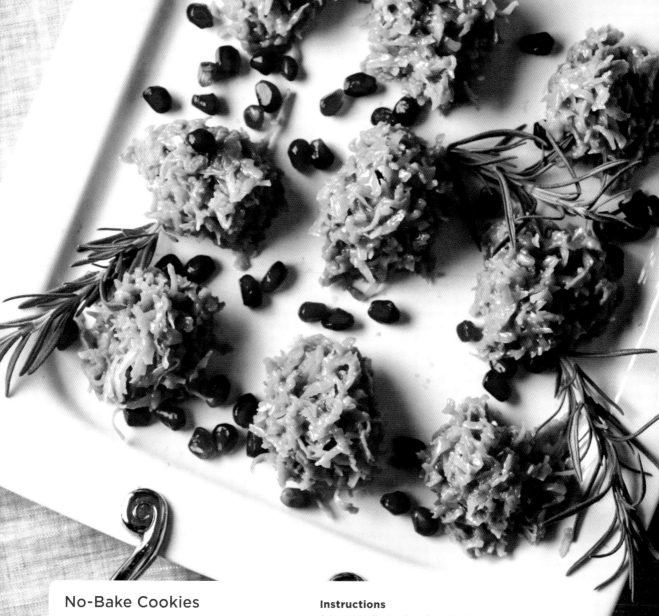

No-Bake Cookies

These peanut butter and coconut treats are simply addictive!

PREP 5 minutes
TOTAL 10 minutes + 5 minutes inactive
SERVINGS 16

Ingredients

- 2 tablespoons butter
- 1 tablespoon stevia
- ⅔ cup all-natural peanut butter
- 1 cup unsweetened shredded coconut
- ½ teaspoon vanilla extract
- Garnishes: pomegranate seeds, rosemary sprigs

Instructions

1 In a medium glass bowl, mix butter and stevia; microwave for 1 minute.

2 Stir in peanut butter. Add coconut and vanilla extract, mixing well.

3 Line a baking sheet with parchment. Spoon tablespoons of the mixture onto prepared baking sheet.

4 Freeze for 5 minutes.

5 Store in the refrigerator until ready to serve; garnish as desired.

NUTRITION INFORMATION (per serving)
Calories: 174; Fat: 16g; Protein: 5g; Carbs: 6g; Fiber: 3g; Net Carbs: 3g

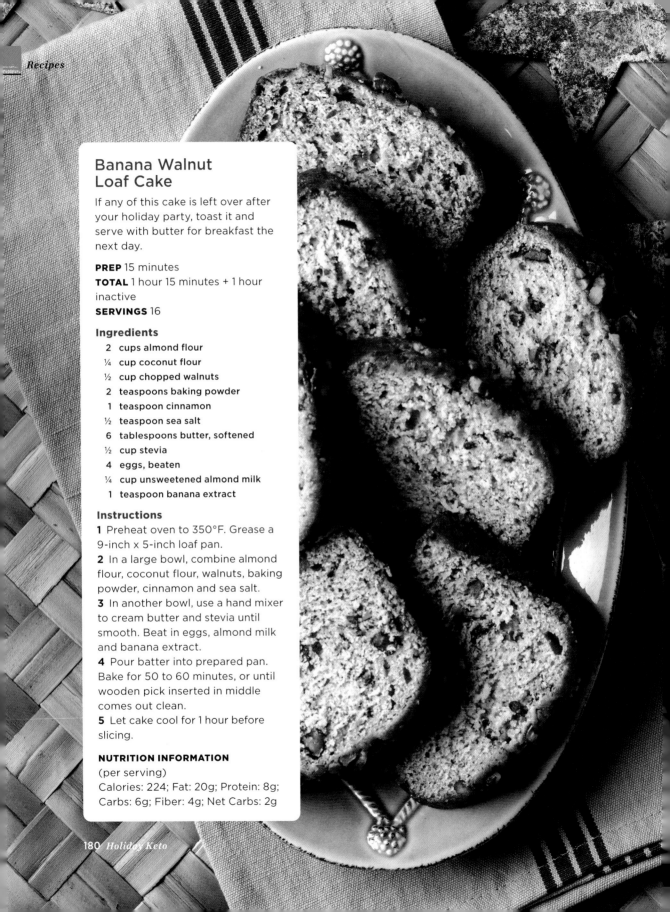

Banana Walnut Loaf Cake

If any of this cake is left over after your holiday party, toast it and serve with butter for breakfast the next day.

PREP 15 minutes
TOTAL 1 hour 15 minutes + 1 hour inactive
SERVINGS 16

Ingredients

- 2 cups almond flour
- ¼ cup coconut flour
- ½ cup chopped walnuts
- 2 teaspoons baking powder
- 1 teaspoon cinnamon
- ½ teaspoon sea salt
- 6 tablespoons butter, softened
- ½ cup stevia
- 4 eggs, beaten
- ¼ cup unsweetened almond milk
- 1 teaspoon banana extract

Instructions

1 Preheat oven to 350°F. Grease a 9-inch x 5-inch loaf pan.
2 In a large bowl, combine almond flour, coconut flour, walnuts, baking powder, cinnamon and sea salt.
3 In another bowl, use a hand mixer to cream butter and stevia until smooth. Beat in eggs, almond milk and banana extract.
4 Pour batter into prepared pan. Bake for 50 to 60 minutes, or until wooden pick inserted in middle comes out clean.
5 Let cake cool for 1 hour before slicing.

NUTRITION INFORMATION

(per serving)
Calories: 224; Fat: 20g; Protein: 8g; Carbs: 6g; Fiber: 4g; Net Carbs: 2g

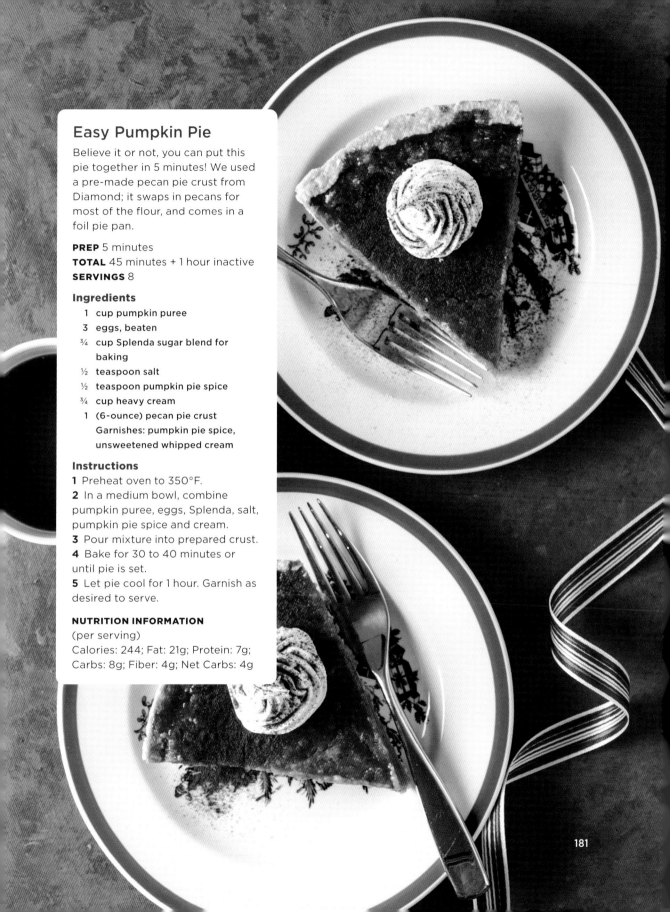

Easy Pumpkin Pie

Believe it or not, you can put this pie together in 5 minutes! We used a pre-made pecan pie crust from Diamond; it swaps in pecans for most of the flour, and comes in a foil pie pan.

PREP 5 minutes
TOTAL 45 minutes + 1 hour inactive
SERVINGS 8

Ingredients

- 1 cup pumpkin puree
- 3 eggs, beaten
- ¾ cup Splenda sugar blend for baking
- ½ teaspoon salt
- ½ teaspoon pumpkin pie spice
- ¾ cup heavy cream
- 1 (6-ounce) pecan pie crust
  Garnishes: pumpkin pie spice, unsweetened whipped cream

Instructions

1 Preheat oven to 350°F.
2 In a medium bowl, combine pumpkin puree, eggs, Splenda, salt, pumpkin pie spice and cream.
3 Pour mixture into prepared crust.
4 Bake for 30 to 40 minutes or until pie is set.
5 Let pie cool for 1 hour. Garnish as desired to serve.

NUTRITION INFORMATION

(per serving)
Calories: 244; Fat: 21g; Protein: 7g; Carbs: 8g; Fiber: 4g; Net Carbs: 4g

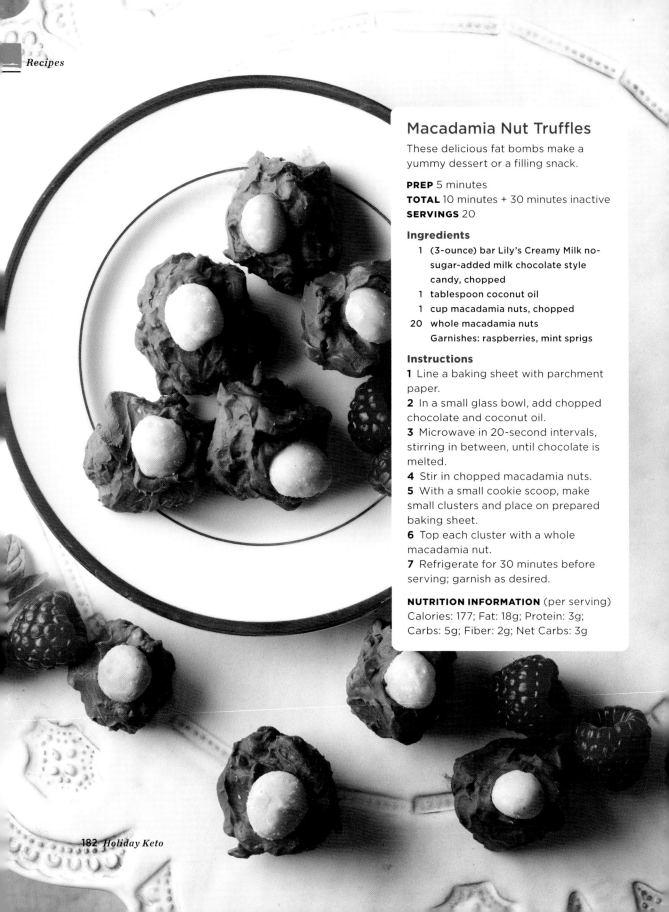

Macadamia Nut Truffles

These delicious fat bombs make a yummy dessert or a filling snack.

PREP 5 minutes
TOTAL 10 minutes + 30 minutes inactive
SERVINGS 20

Ingredients

- 1 (3-ounce) bar Lily's Creamy Milk no-sugar-added milk chocolate style candy, chopped
- 1 tablespoon coconut oil
- 1 cup macadamia nuts, chopped
- 20 whole macadamia nuts
  Garnishes: raspberries, mint sprigs

Instructions

1 Line a baking sheet with parchment paper.
2 In a small glass bowl, add chopped chocolate and coconut oil.
3 Microwave in 20-second intervals, stirring in between, until chocolate is melted.
4 Stir in chopped macadamia nuts.
5 With a small cookie scoop, make small clusters and place on prepared baking sheet.
6 Top each cluster with a whole macadamia nut.
7 Refrigerate for 30 minutes before serving; garnish as desired.

NUTRITION INFORMATION (per serving)
Calories: 177; Fat: 18g; Protein: 3g; Carbs: 5g; Fiber: 2g; Net Carbs: 3g

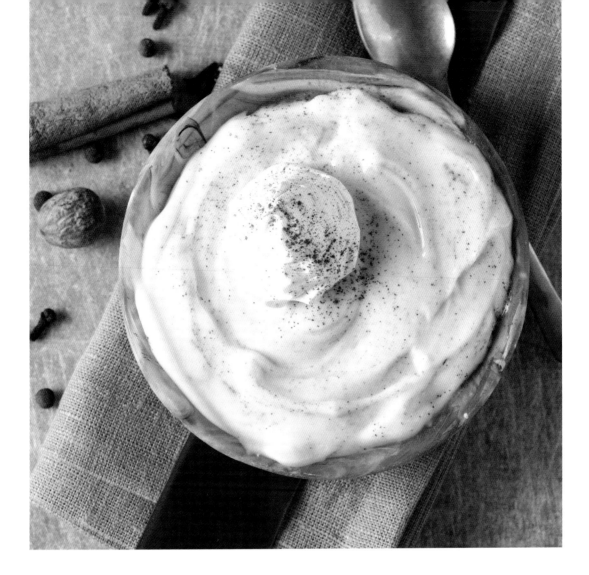

Pumpkin Pie Pudding

Substitute any flavorings you like in place of the pumpkin pie spice.

PREP 25 minutes
TOTAL 90 minutes
SERVINGS 6

Ingredients

- 1   tablespoon stevia
- 1   teaspoon pumpkin pie spice
- ⅛   teaspoon xanthan gum
- 1   teaspoon vanilla
- 1   cup heavy cream
- ½   cup coconut milk
- 3   egg whites
    Garnishes: whipped cream, pumpkin pie spice

Instructions

1 In a mixing bowl, combine stevia, pumpkin pie spice and xanthan gum.
2 Add vanilla, cream, coconut milk and egg whites.
3 Beat with a hand mixer on high for 3 minutes.
4 Pour the mixture into a saucepan and heat over medium-high heat. Stir constantly for 3 minutes.
5 Transfer pudding to individual dessert bowls; cool to room temperature for 15 minutes.
6 Refrigerate pudding for 1 hour. Garnish as desired to serve.

NUTRITION INFORMATION (per serving)
Calories: 325; Fat: 25g; Protein: 4.5g; Carbs: 4g; Fiber: 1g; Net Carbs: 3g

No-Bake Chocolate Torte

Use a high quality of sugar-free unsweetened chocolate in this treat.

PREP 5 minutes
TOTAL 15 minutes + 1 hour inactive
SERVINGS 12

Ingredients

- 1¼ cups heavy cream
- ¼ cup stevia
- 2 (3.5-ounce) bars unsweetened chocolate, chopped
- 7 tablespoons butter
- ¾ cup walnuts, chopped and toasted
- ¼ cup pumpkin seeds, toasted
- ⅛ teaspoon sea salt
- Garnishes: flaky sea salt, chopped walnuts, raspberries, mint leaves

Instructions

1 In a saucepan, bring cream and stevia to a boil. Reduce heat; simmer for 3 minutes or until creamy. Remove from heat.

2 Stir in the chopped chocolate and butter until melted and combined.

3 Stir in the chopped walnuts and the pumpkin seeds.

4 Grease an 8-inch springform pan; spoon mixture into pan and sprinkle with sea salt.

5 Cover and refrigerate torte for 1 hour or until hardened.

6 Place torte on platter, and garnish as desired to serve.

NUTRITION INFORMATION (per serving)
Calories: 215; Fat: 21g; Protein: 5g; Carbs: 4g; Fiber: 2g; Net Carbs: 2g

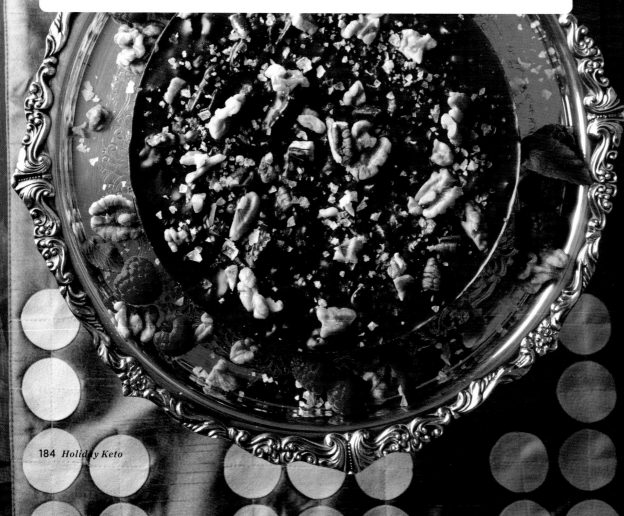

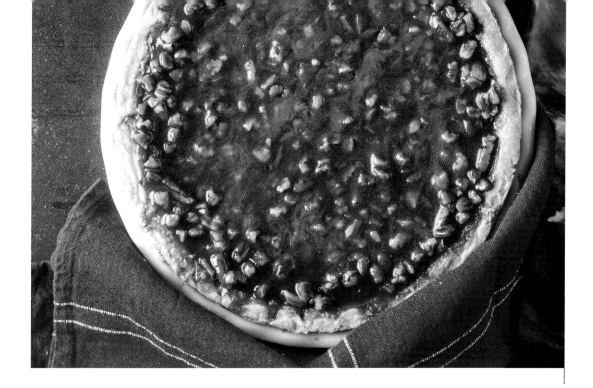

Pecan Pie

Just as sweet, gooey and tasty as the original!

PREP 40 minutes
TOTAL 1 hour 20 minutes + 1 hour 35 minutes inactive
SERVINGS 10

Ingredients

- 2 cups almond flour
- 2 teaspoons powdered monk fruit sweetener
- 1 teaspoon sea salt
- ⅓ cup butter
- 2 tablespoons coconut oil
- 4 large eggs
- 1 cup butter
- 1 cup golden monk fruit sweetener
- 2 tablespoons almond butter
- 1 cup canned coconut milk
- 2 teaspoons vanilla extract
- 2½ cups chopped pecans

Instructions

1 Preheat oven to 325°F.

2 In a food processor, combine almond flour, powdered sweetener, ½ teaspoon sea salt, butter and coconut oil. Pulse until mixture forms pea-size crumbs.

3 Add 1 egg; pulse until dough comes together.

Add more almond flour as needed if dough seems too wet.

4 Form dough into a ball and wrap in plastic wrap; chill in refrigerator for 20 minutes.

5 Place dough between 2 sheets of parchment paper; roll into a large circle.

6 Lay dough round over a 9-inch pie dish and press into the bottom and up sides of the dish. Trim and flute edges.

7 Place pie dish in the freezer for 10 minutes.

8 Meanwhile, in heavy-bottomed saucepan over medium heat, melt butter, stirring constantly.

9 Remove saucepan from heat; whisk in golden sweetener, almond butter, coconut milk, remaining ½ teaspoon sea salt and vanilla extract until smooth. Cool for 5 minutes.

10 In a small bowl, beat remaining 3 eggs. Slowly whisk them into coconut milk mixture until combined. Stir in chopped pecans.

11 Pour mixture into prepared pie crust.

12 Bake for 40 to 45 minutes or until the center is nearly set and the crust is deep golden brown. Cover crust with foil to prevent over-browning, if needed.

13 Let pie cool for at least 1 hour before serving.

NUTRITION INFORMATION (per serving)
Calories: 425; Fat: 46g; Protein: 8g; Carbs: 8g; Fiber: 4g; Net Carbs: 4g

A

Abdominal fat, 24
Above-ground vegetables, 34
Accomplishments, recognizing own, 96
Acetone, 47
Alcohol
   in keto diet, 58
   keto-friendly beverage recipes, 120–129
   setting up a bar with, 112–113
Alternate-day fasting, 53
Antioxidants, in low-carb vegetables, 42–43
Appetizers, 130–139
   quantity per person, 116
Arugula Salad With Feta and Cranberries, 143
Asparagus Salad With Pistachios, 146
Avocado oil, 37

B

Bacon and Cauliflower Soup, 149
Bacon-Wrapped Asparagus, 131
Bad breath, 47
Baked Salmon With Lemon and Herbs, 161
Baking ingredients, keto-friendly, 40–41
Banana Walnut Loaf Cake, 180
Bar, tips on setting up, 112–113
Basics of keto, 6–59
BBG (DVD), 90
Beef jerky, 77
Beef Tenderloin With Horseradish Cream, 160
Bell peppers, 42
Below-ground vegetables, 34
"Belly" fat, 24
Berries, 40
Beverages
   recipes, 120–129
   serving tips, 112–113
Bikini Body Guide (*BBG*) DVD series, 90
Blood glucose/sugar, 24, 26, 34, 52
Body, overall keto benefits for, 27
Bourbon Baked Ham, 164
Brain function, 22–23, 27
Breakfast, skipping, 90
Broccoli, 42
Broccoli Cheddar Soup, 153
Brussels Sprout Casserole, 173
Buffet, tips on setting up, 108–109
Butter Pecan Cheesecake, 178

C

Cancer, keto benefits for, 25
Canned fish, 77
Caramelized Onion Dip, 132
Carb cravings, 46, 48–49
   coping strategies, 82–85
   food swaps for, 49, 84–85
Carb cycling, 52, 77, 80
"Carb day," 74
   exercise on, 81
Carbohydrates, 52. *See also* Carb *entries*
   compared, 34
   fats *vs.*, 28–35
   good vs. bad, 34–35
   insulin and, 17–18
   ratio in keto diet, 19
   in vegetables, 34–35
Celebrations. *See* Party season, keto-friendly
   strategies during
Celery, 43
Champagne, 58
Charcuterie, 77
Cheats, good and bad, 85
Cheese, 40, 77
   handling, 109
Chicharróns (pork rinds), 77
Chicken and Cauliflower Rice Soup, 152
Chocolate Peppermint Cocktail, 121
Cholesterol
   HDL, 52
   LDL, 53
Cocktails
   recipes, 120–129
   serving tips, 112–113
Coconut oil, 37
Cold-pressed oils, 37
Commitment, to keto diet
   during holiday season, 66–67
   maintenance strategy, 57
Compound exercise moves, 88
Constipation, 47, 104
Contributions, to holiday/celebratory event, 66
Corn Chowder, 148
Cranberry Mimosa, 127
Cranberry Mousse, 177
Cranberry Sauce, 172
Cranberry Vodka Spritzer, 121

Cravings. *See* Carb cravings
Cream of Asparagus Soup, 154
Creamed Spinach With Nutmeg, 174
Creamy Blue Cheese Dip With Chicken Wings, 138
Creamy Mushrooms With Thyme, 167
Cucumbers, 43
"Cycle" day, 80
    exercise on, 81

D

Dairy products, 40
Decorations, natural, 110–111
Deep-breathing exercise, 97
Desserts, 176–185
    quantity per person, 117
    separate buffet table for, 109
Diabetes, type 2, 30
Dietary restrictions, speaking up about, 65–66, 70
"Dirty" keto, 52
Drinks (alcoholic)
    recipes, 120–129
    serving tips, 112–113
DVDs, for at-home exercise routine, 90

E

Easy Pumpkin Pie, 181
Eating
    alcohol and, 58
    exercise before, 90
    on the go, best keto-friendly foods for, 76, 77
    keto cycling and, 78–81
    mindfulness when, 97
    when tired, 101
Eggnog Martini, 128
Eggplant and Tomato Stacks With Rosemary, 144
Eggs, 40
Electrolytes, 52, 104
Entertaining, stress-free, 106–117
    beverage bar, 112–113
    buffets, 108–109
    decorations, 110–111
    food quantities per person, 116–117
    holiday dinner time line, 114–115
Entrées
    quantity per person, 117
    recipes, 156–165

Exercise
    aerobic workouts, 88, 90
    at-home routines, 90
    on "carb" days, 81
    compound moves, 88
    in daily routine, 88
    early in day, 90
    enjoyable, 96
Exercise plans, for holiday season, 86–91
Exogenous ketones, 52

F

Fasting, intermittent, 53
Fat(s), 18
    in brain, 23
    carbs *vs.*, 28–35
    compared, 31–34
    good vs. bad, 34–35
    key keto facts, 15
    ratio in keto diet, 19
Fish
    canned, 77
    as protein source, 41
Flours, keto-friendly, 40–41
Food processor, 57
Food scale, 57
Food spiralizer, 57
Food swaps, in carb-heavy meals, 49, 84–85
Food(s)
    low-carb, 40–41
    portion sizes, 116–117
    pre-portioning for buffet, 109
    processed, 30
    relationship with, reevaluating, 94, 96
    when traveling, 76, 77
Fruits, key keto facts about, 15

G

Garlic, 42
Ghrelin, 100
Glucose/Glycogen, 52
Goals, setting, 92–97
Greek yogurt, 40
Green beans, 43
Group support, 95
Gut health, keto benefits for, 27

H

Habits, understanding own, 66

Hard liquor, 58

HDL cholesterol, 23, 52

Healthfulness, of keto diet, 14

Heart-health outcomes, 23–24, 27

Heavy-duty food processor, 57

High-fat–low-carb regimen. *See* Ketogenic diet/
  lifestyle

High-intensity interval training (HIIT), 88, 90

Holiday dinner
  preparation time line, 114–115
  quantity per person, 116–117

Holiday gatherings. *See* Party season, keto-
  friendly strategies during

Holiday Salad With Tomatoes and Avocado, 141

Holiday season
  dining away from home in, 72–75
  exercise plans for, 86–91
  parties during. *See* Party season, keto-friendly
    strategies during

Holiday Vodka Chata, 124

Homemade Ranch Dip With Assorted Vegetables,
  139

Hosting tips, 106–117. *See also* Entertaining,
  stress-free

Hosts, communicating with, 66, 70

Hot Buttered Rum, 126

Hot Chocolate, 122

Hydration, 102–105

Hydration equation, 104

I

Insulin, 17–18, 34, 52

Intermittent fasting, 53

Inulin, 52–53

Italian Antipasto Salad, 142

Italian Sausage Stuffed Mushrooms, 135

J

Joints, keto benefits for, 27

K

Kale Salad With Goat Cheese and Pomegranate
  Seeds, 145

Keto cycling plan, 78–81. *See also* Carb cycling

Keto flu, 47, 53, 104

Ketogenic diet/lifestyle
  basics of, 6–59
  defined, 53
  family pushback on, coping with, 70–71
  getting started on, 54–57
  glossary, 52–53
  goals and tactics for, 94–97
  hidden benefits of, 20–27
  maintaining. *See* Planning, for maintaining
    healthy lifestyle
  preferred foods in, 40–41
  science of, 16–17
  seasonal strategies, 60–117. *See also* Party
    season, keto-friendly strategies during
  side effects of, 47

Ketones, 22, 53
  exogenous, 52

Ketosis
  defined, 53
  keto cycle plan and, 80–81. *See also* Carb cycling
  oils and, 36–37
  testing for, 52

Kitchen equipment, 57

Kitchen pantry, reorganizing/stocking, 57

L

Labeling buffet dishes, 109

Lamb, Leg of, With Root Vegetables, 162

LDL cholesterol, 24, 53

Leafy greens, 42

Leftover Turkey Chowder, 150

Leg cramps, 47–48

Leptin, 100

Lincoln, Abraham, 57

Liquor, hard, 58

Low-carb diets
  compared with keto, 31
  high-fat regimens and, 31
  low-fat diets *vs.*, 24

Low-carb foods, 40–43

Low-fat diets
  consequences of, 30
  low-carb diets *vs.*, 24
  weight loss and, 31

Lungs, keto benefits for, 27

M

Macadamia nut oil, 37
Macadamia Nut Truffles, 182
"Mac" and Cheese, 171
Macronutrients (macros), 53
  ratios, 19
Magnesium, 104
Main dishes
  quantity per person, 117
  recipes, 156–165
Mantras, 96
MCT oil, 53, 76
Melatonin, 101
Metabolism, keto benefits for, 26
Mindfulness strategies, 97
Mini Cheese Truffles, 136
Motivation, re-affirming, 66–67
Movement, incorporating in daily routine, 88
Mulled wine, 123
Multitasking, avoiding, 97

N

National Institutes of Health, sleep amount
    recommendations, 100
National Sleep Foundation, 100, 101
Natural decorations, 110–111
No-Bake Chocolate Torte, 184
No-Bake Cookies, 179
Noon, exercise before, 90
Nut butters, 41, 77
Nuts, 41, 77

O

Obesity epidemic, 30
Oils. *See also individual oils*
  ketosis and, 36–37
  MCT (supplement), 53, 76
Olive oil, 33, 35, 37, 76
Olives, 77
Omega-3 fatty acids, 33, 34, 77
Onion, 43

P

Pantry, reorganization/stocking, 57
Party season, keto-friendly strategies during,
    62–67
  cycle plan for, 78–81

eating out, 72–77
exercise and, 86–91
hydration and, 102–105
planning ahead for, 68–71
rule breaking and, 82–85
setting goals, 92–97
sleep and, 98–101
Patience, 96
Pecan Pie, 185
Periodic fasting, 53
Pilates Intense Interval Training (*PIIT 28*) DVD,
    90
Pistachio-Crusted Chicken Breasts, 165
Planning, for maintaining healthy lifestyle
  coping strategies for carb cravings, 85
  dining away from home, 72–77
  eating on the go, best keto-friendly foods for, 76,
      77
  during party season, 68–71
Polycystic ovarian syndrome (PCOS), keto
    benefits for, 25–26
Pork Chops With Pesto, 157
Pork rinds, 77
Pork Tenderloin With Mustard Sauce, 158
Portion sizes, 116–117
  pre-portioning and, 109
Potassium, 104
Prebiotic, defined, 53
Pre-portioning, 109
Processed foods, 30
Protein
  food choices for, 41
  key keto facts, 15
  ratio in keto diet, 19
Pumpkin Pie Pudding, 183
Pumpkin Spice Latter, 129

Q

Quick "cheats," good and bad, 85

R

Raspberry Moscow Mule, 125
Recipes
  appetizers, 130–139
  beverages, 120–129
  desserts, 176–185
  entrées, 156–165

salads, 140–147
    side dishes, 166–175
    soups, 148–155
Reframing strategy, 65
Restaurant menus, navigating, 65, 76
Roasted Brussels Sprouts With Garlic Aioli, 137
Roasted Butternut Squash Soup, 151
Roasted Turkey Breast With Vegetables, 159
Roasted Vegetable Salad, 147

S
Salads, 140–147
Saturated fat, 33
Sautéed Cabbage With Bacon, 175
Savory Sage Stuffing, 167
Science of keto diet, 16–17
Seafood. *See* Fish
Seasonal strategies, 60–117. *See also* Party season,
    keto-friendly strategies during
Seeds, 41
Sesame Broccoli, 170
Sesame oil, 37
Shellfish, 41
Shopping list, 59
Shopping strategy, 57
Shrimp With Spicy Remoulade, 134
Side dishes, 166–175
    quantity per person, 117
Skin, keto benefits for, 27
Sleep, 98–101
    recommended amount, 100
    tips on, 100–101
Sleep deprivation, 100
Sleep experience, 101
Slow-Cooked Beef Brisket, 163
Sodium, 104
Soup recipes, 148–155
Spiced Vanilla Cake, 177
Spicy Pimento Cheese With Pecans, 133
Spinach Dip With Parmesan Crisps, 131
Spinach Salad With Eggs and Bacon, 141
Spiralizer, 57
Squat breaks, 8
Stretches, 88
Sugar cravings. *See* Carb cravings
Supplements
    exogenous ketones, 52

    liquid electrolytes, 104
    MCT oil, 53

T
Tendencies, understanding own, 66
Time-restricted feeding, 53
Tired, eating when, 101
Traveling, packing own food for, 76, 77
Triggers, carb cravings and, 84
Triglycerides, 53
    MCT oil, 53
Turkey, cooking time for, 114
Turkey Sausage and Kale Soup, 155

U
Unsaturated fat, 34

V
Vegetables
    carbs in, 34–35
    key keto facts about, 15
    low-carb, 41–43
    prebiotic content in, 53

W
Warm Kale With Gorgonzola, 168
Water, in transition to keto diet, 102–105
Weight fluctuations, on carb/cycle days, 81
Weight loss, 18, 21
    drinking water and, 103–104
Whipped Cauliflower Mash, 169
Whole Roasted Chicken With Radishes, 157
Wine, 58

Y
Yawning exercise, 97

Z
"Zoodles" (zucchini noodles), 57

CREDITS

COVER Pinkyone/Shutterstock (Bow) stacy2010ua/Shutterstock **FRONT FLAP** Liam Franklin/Recipe styling and development: Margaret Monroe **1** Pinkyone/Shutterstock **2-4** Liam Franklin/Recipe styling and development: Margaret Monroe (2) **5** (From left) laflor/Getty Images; PeopleImages/Getty Images; Liam Franklin/Recipe styling and development: Margaret Monroe **6-7** Eva-Katalin/Getty Images **8** The Picture Pantry/Lisovskaya Na/Getty Images **10** Claudia Totir/Getty Images **11** (Clockwise from top left) alle12/Getty Images; Johanna Parkin/Getty Images; Creativ Studio Heinemann/Getty Images; LordRunar/Getty Images; VMJones/Getty Images; JazzIRT/Getty Images **12-13** Maskot/Getty Images **15** (Clockwise from top) Jurgen Magg/Getty Images; Floortje/Getty Images; marius FM77/Getty Images **16-17** laflor/Getty Images **19** (Clockwise from top left) Artem Varnitsin/EyeEm/Getty Images; Westend61/Getty Images; mashuk/iStockphoto/Getty Images; PeopleImages/Getty Images; Frank Bean/Uppercut RF/Getty Images (2); Photo by Cathy Scola/Getty Images; EasyBuy4u/Getty Images; Lew Robertson/Getty Images **20** Erik Dreyer/Getty Images **22-23** caia image/Alamy Stock Photo **25** wildpixel/Getty Images **26** PhotoAlto/Frederic Cirou/Getty Images **27** Tara Moore/Getty Images **28** Flavia Morlachetti/Getty Images **29** Foodcollection RF/Getty Images **30** (From left) AlasdairJames/Getty Images; Francesco Perre/EyeEm/Getty Images; Les Weber/EyeEm/Getty Images **31** (From left) Floortje/Getty Images; William Turner/Getty Images; John E. Kelly/Getty Images **32-33** Tim Macpherson/Getty Images **35** (Clockwise from top left) the_burtons/Getty Images; Anna-Ok/Getty Images; Amarita/Getty Images; MakiEni's photo/Getty Images **36** Sunny/Getty Images **37** William Turner/Getty Images **38-39** Rodica Ciorba/Getty Images **40-41** istetiana/Getty Images **42** (From left) mahirart/Shutterstock; Maks Narodenko/Shutterstock; Nattika/Shutterstock; Nik Merkulov/Shutterstock **43** (Clockwise from left) Tim UR/Shutterstock; Bozena Fulawka/Shutterstock; Anna Sedneva/Shutterstock; MRS.Siwaporn/Shutterstock **44** Terry Vine/Getty Images **46** Orbon Alija/Getty Images **48** JGI/Jamie Grill/Getty Images **49** (Background) kyoshino/Getty Images (Clockwise from top right) photominer/Shutterstock; Has Asatryan/Shutterstock; asife/Shutterstock; Westend61/Getty Images; boblin/Getty Images; Creative Crop/Getty Images; Science Photo Library/Getty Images; Maren Caruso/Getty Images; Annabelle Breakey/Getty Images; Manny Rodriguez/Getty Images; Jacqueline Han/EyeEm/Getty Images; Oran Tantapakul/EyeEm/Getty Images **50** GlobalStock/Getty Images **52** AndreyPopov/Getty Images **53** vasiliybudarin/Getty Images **54-55** ZUKAGAWA/Getty Images **56** SDI Productions/Getty Images **58** mapodile/Getty Images **59** (From top) Julia Filipenko/Shutterstock; Armin Staudt/EyeEm/Getty Images; Floortje/Getty Images **60-61** sergio_kumer/Getty Images **62-63** lisegagne/Getty Images **64-65** Prostock-Studio/Getty Images **67** skynesher/Getty Images **68** andresr/Getty Images **70-71** PeopleImages/Getty Images **72-73** Photographee.eu/Shutterstock **74-75** Alexander Spatari/Getty Images **77** Lew Robertson/Getty Images **78-79** Westend61/Getty Images **80-81** LightFieldStudios/Getty Images **82-83** Image Source/Getty Images **84-85** Mizina/Getty Images **86-89** PeopleImages/Getty Images (2) **91** Maskot/Getty Images **92** WillSelarep/Getty Images **94-95** vitranc/Getty Images **97** PeopleImages/Getty Images **98-99** StoryTime Studio/Shutterstock **100** AndreyPopov/Getty Images **101** PeopleImages/Getty Images **102-103** Halfpoint/Shutterstock **105** kraftstock/Getty Images **106-107** Britany George/EyeEm/Getty Images **108-109** emmaduckworth/RooM RF/Getty Images **110** Lina Östling/Folio/Getty Images **111** (Center) Anfisa Kameneva/EyeEm/Getty Images (Clockwise from top left) Sally Williams Photography/Getty Images; John Block/Getty Images; Alexandra Grablewski/Getty Images; Claudia Totir/Getty Images; Lina √ñstling/Folio Images RF/Getty Images; Juliette Wade/Getty Images; emmaduckworth/RooM RF/Getty Images; Annabelle Breakey/Getty Images **112** NightAndDayImages/Getty Images **113** wmaster890/Getty Images **114** Edalin/Getty Images **115** Carol Yepes/Getty Images **116** Tatiana Volgutova/Getty Images **117** (Clockwise from top) grandriver/Getty Images; LauriPatterson/Getty Images; haoliang/Getty Images **118-185** Liam Franklin/Recipe styling and development: Margaret Monroe (67) **SPINE** stacy2010ua/Shutterstock **BACK FLAP, BACK COVER** Liam Franklin/Recipe styling and development: Margaret Monroe (13)

Special thanks to contributing writers:
Nancy Coulter-Parker, Margaret Monroe, Shari Goldhagen, Stacy Baker Masand, Caroline McKenzie and Joanna Powell

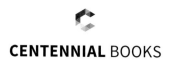

CENTENNIAL BOOKS

An Imprint of
Centennial Media, LLC
40 Worth St., 10th Floor
New York, NY 10013, U.S.A.

CENTENNIAL BOOKS is a trademark of Centennial Media, LLC

ISBN 978-1-951274-45-0

Distributed by
Simon & Schuster, Inc.
1230 Avenue of the Americas
New York, NY 10020, U.S.A.

For information about custom editions, special sales and premium and corporate purchases,
please contact Centennial Media at contact@centennialmedia.com.

Manufactured in China

10 9 8 7 6 5 4 3 2 1

Publishers & Co-Founders Ben Harris, Sebastian Raatz
Editorial Director Annabel Vered
Creative Director Jessica Power
Executive Editor Janet Giovanelli
Deputy Editors Ron Kelly, Alyssa Shaffer
Design Director Ben Margherita
Art Directors Andrea Lukeman,
Natali Suasnavas, Joseph Ulatowski
Assistant Art Director Jaclyn Loney
Photo Editor Kim Kuhn
Production Manager Paul Rodina
Production Assistant Alyssa Swiderski
Editorial Assistant Tiana Schippa
Sales & Marketing Jeremy Nurnberg